WITH LOVE

Jerry

4 PATHS OF
CANCER

A Journey Through Myths, Grief, Hope, Love

Terry Novak, RN

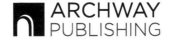
ARCHWAY
PUBLISHING

Archway Publishing books may be ordered through booksellers or by contacting:

Archway Publishing
1663 Liberty Drive
Bloomington, IN 47403
www.archwaypublishing.com
844-669-3957

ISBN: 978-1-6657-4559-8 (sc)
ISBN: 978-1-6657-4560-4 (e)

Library of Congress Control Number: 2023911166

Print information available on the last page.

Archway Publishing rev. date: 09/20/2023

There is no traced-out path to lead man to his salvation; he must constantly invent his own path. But, to invent it, he is free, responsible, without excuse, and every hope lies within him.

—Sartre, philosopher of existentialism

To all the patients, family members, loved ones, and health care professionals who have made and are still making this journey. Thank you.

CONTENTS

ACKNOWLEDGMENTS

First of all, Ron, my life partner of over twenty-five years. He has believed in me when I didn't believe in myself. He encouraged me when I wasn't sure I could take another step. He has been my soft place to fall. He makes me laugh. He always makes sure I and our fur babies are taken care of and safe.

Second, Cyndi, who came into my life when she was a scared teenage girl at a crossroads in her life as well as mine. Over thirty years later and now a proud mother and grandmother, she is still in my life. She gave me and taught me as much as I hope I gave and taught her through these years. She inspires me every day with her strength, courage, integrity, commitment to her family, and laughter. She is my "adopted" daughter. She was the beautiful gift I needed most in my life.

I must be honest. I knew nothing about being a cancer research nurse when I was hired. My mom had died of lymphoma, but I really didn't understand the depth of the disease beyond knowing it was a blood cancer. I wonder if I had known then what I know now if I could have done more for her.

Fortunately, when I started, I worked with two amazing people: an oncologist, Dr. Claire Verschraegen (Dr. V), and a lab tech for the clinical trials, Elsie Wilson. They patiently guided me and taught me how to be a research nurse, how to hold myself to a higher standard, to see the patient as a human being and not just the disease afflicting a patient (such a sterile name, *patient*). Gradually, I learned how to become an advocate for the person in front of me, to be their voice when their own voice was silenced by fear of yet another unknown—not just the unknown of cancer but the unknown of a potential new drug that might or might not benefit them but could possibly benefit someone in the future, the fear of their own unknown future, the fear of their own mortality. I took this responsibility seriously, dutifully, and gratefully.

Dr. V is the MacGyver of oncologists. She could always find a way to make something happen that needed to happen. She is tenacious, fearless, compassionate, and creative. She loves her patients.

Elsie is Navajo and a beautiful soul. She epitomizes the meaning of the Navajo word *hozro*: the blend of being in harmony with one's environment, at peace with one's circumstances, content with the day, devoid of anger, and free from anxiety. She brought this spirit to all her patients and staff who worked with her. Patients loved her. She always got the blood draw on the first stick! She would let me know if something didn't feel right with a patient. She had a sixth sense about people, especially the depth of their silent suffering.

Dr. Montaser (Monte) Shaheen followed Dr. V as the phase 1 clinical trials researcher. He became my mentor, teaching me more about research and the importance of clinical trials in developing new treatments, especially for the most difficult cancers. He also became my dear friend. He takes his extensive knowledge of cancer genetics, epigenetics, and genomics and applies it to real patients in the real world, not just the lab. He lives in possibility, outside the clinical box.

Dr. Arpit Rao was a second-year oncology fellow when I met him. He joined our phase 1 research team during the last six months of his fellowship. He is a combination of intelligence, compassion, and vision. He was my confidante, friend, and a natural researcher and tireless clinician. It was a pleasure and an honor to work with him. I never worried about a patient in his care.

Last, but not least, I would like to thank all the patients who entrusted me with their care and who so unselfishly gave the gift of hope to others they would never know but who would follow them. They will always live in my heart.

Please, if you're a nurse, love details and being on the cutting edge of science, and want to spend more quality and unforgettable time with your patients, consider becoming a research nurse. It will change your life and maybe the lives of your patients.

I truly believe the right opportunities and the right people come into our lives at exactly the right time and in exactly the right way. I will be forever grateful these people and these opportunities came into my life when they did. They continue to shape my life.

> *In the sweetness of friendship let there be laughter, and*
> *sharing of pleasures. For in the dew of little things the heart*
> *finds its morning and is refreshed.*
> —*Kahlil Gibran, author of The Prophet*

INTRODUCTION

Life is what happens when you're busy making other plans.
—John Lennon

PURPOSE

My intention in writing this book is not to offer scientific or medical advice, explanations, or recommendations about diagnoses or treatments. My intention, my hope, is to destigmatize, demystify, and humanize cancer so that patients, families, friends, and caregivers can be with the diagnosis in a way that is empowering for everyone and not see it first as a hopeless death sentence or a new definition of who the patient is. The cancer of today is a different disease, with newer, more effective treatments that have less-destructive side effects. It is my belief, my hope, that cancer will become a manageable chronic disease, like heart disease or diabetes, and that people will be able to live with it and have a good quality of life.

What I have written is based on my own personal and professional observations and interactions with clinical trial patients as a cancer research nurse of almost ten years, and from friends and family members diagnosed and living with or dying from cancer. These are the lessons they have taught me and the blessings they have shared with me. I am forever grateful.

No one wants to hear a doctor say, "You have cancer." Such an ugly word. It sucks the very air out of the room when it's spoken. Everything becomes silent, and time stops. You think or say things like, *Wait, not me. It can't be. That happens to someone else. I'm too young. It's just a cough. I'm too healthy. I've done everything right. No one in my family has had cancer. I have so much left to do. Am I going to die?*

Cancer is impersonal, relentless, undiplomatic, unsympathetic, unforgiving, unfair, merciless, unloving, mysterious, invasive, treacherous, serendipitous, fortuitous, guerrilla-like, ambitious, depleting, conquerable, detectable, manageable, treatable, silent, frightening, promising, honorable, memorable, competitive, bloodsucking, survivable, reinventing, nauseating, gift-giving, complicated, unpredictable, undeniable, divisive, unifying, challenging, draining, and overwhelming, and it requires that you embrace it all moment to moment, sometimes all at once.

No one else, even someone with cancer or a survivor of cancer, will ever fully understand what it means to *you* to have cancer—no matter how hard they try or think they do. You and your experiences are unique to you. There may be similarities and some common ground, but no one else can feel it the way you do. This is your own journey, with rest stops along the way and people willing to take you in without judgment. Other people will never completely understand what you're experiencing, but they will try to see you, hear you, and love you as best they can. Those are the most embraceable parts.

My hope is to be a Sherpa for you on this journey as you traverse the depths and the heights, all the unknowns, the chasms, the falls, and the unexpected. You are not alone, even in your darkest times. There is hope and even love to be found on this journey. Impossible? *No.*

My hopes and intentions are to empower you, your family, and your loved ones as you journey through your cancer diagnosis, treatments, and last days, if that's the eventual outcome. Cancer doesn't have to be paralyzing. You don't have to be a *victim* of cancer, and you can be more than a *survivor*. You can live your life; it may be different than before, but you don't have to be defined by cancer.

Attitude is a choice. You have choices, and you have your own inner power and wisdom. There will be difficult, life-changing challenges for everyone. Cancer is a terrible disease. But as more light is shined upon it, the less darkness there is, and that open place of possibility is what I want all those affected to find.

On this journey, we will explore what I call the four paths of cancer based on my own experiences personally and professionally: myths, grief, hope, and love. Simple words, but very complex concepts. I have traveled these paths myself, with patients, their loved ones, my own loved ones, and the amazing health care providers who have dedicated their lives to delivering better care and newer treatments to ease the burden of cancer and provide more-hopeful outcomes, a better quality of life, and a more-promising future. It's not easy for anyone, but it is possible. Every day, new possibilities and new hopes are discovered.

BACKGROUND

I became a registered nurse (RN) in 1977 at the age of twenty-eight—a little older than most nursing students at the time. My first job was in the burn unit of a major hospital and trauma center. This was my first choice for employment. I had been impressed by the unit director, an RN who was also a Sisters of Mercy nun. She spoke at our senior class about job opportunities in her unit. I was immediately struck by her level of compassion and commitment to those suffering patients.

Although a burn unit may sound like a horrible place to work, it was actually very challenging in the most positive way. The patients were usually in the unit a very long time if they didn't die soon after their injuries. We worked very closely with the patients, encouraging them through the most painful of procedures, offering them hope that they would learn to accept their disfigurement and could live a new, though different, life. We also got to know the family members and offered them encouragement and hope that they would get through the challenges that would be facing them, but knowing the odds at the time were not in their favor.

After two years, I became burned out (no pun intended), shutting down all feeling I once had. I knew it was time to move on. I didn't want to be a nurse just going through the motions, no longer able to see the human being inside the patient. I transferred to the level 1 trauma center of this same hospital. Again, this may not sound like a warm and fuzzy place to work. Like the burn unit, it was challenging, but here our patients were with us usually a very short time—just long enough to either be cared for and discharged or stabilized and transferred to the operating room (OR), the intensive care unit (ICU), or the hospital floor; otherwise, they were, unfortunately, dead on arrival (DOA).

It was a different kind of intensity. It was also a place of hope. If the patient was seriously injured or ill, we offered hope to the family that we were doing everything possible to help their loved one. If the patient died, we offered reassurance that their loved one had not suffered while in our care.

After another two years, and it was again time to make a change. By this time, my personal and professional feelings had become deeply buried. I was earning about $12,000 a year, barely enough to support myself, working nights, weekends, and holidays. I had to make a change. I was always looking for something more challenging, new connections, a place where I could feel accepted and appreciated for what I had to offer, and the opportunity to make a livable salary with normal working hours.

Exciting new medical technology was being developed at this time. I was recruited to become a medical sales specialist and be part of bringing this new technology to doctors, clinics, and hospitals. Although not working directly with patients every day, I still had the opportunity to be there with the doctor when he explained how this new equipment or treatment might benefit the patients and once again give them hope. I felt like I was contributing something of value.

I stayed in medical-equipment sales for twenty years. I had my own company for ten of those years. In 2006, I decided to go back to nursing. I wanted to be part of something bigger than myself, something more meaningful, and I wanted to try to give back in a more challenging and measurable way. I completed an RN refresher program so I would be up to speed with all the changes that had occurred while I was in the sales profession. A lot had changed. Nurses had more responsibility, more independence, more autonomy, a bigger voice in patient care, and more career opportunities.

My first position was as a kidney-transplant coordinator. The patients had some form of kidney failure, either chronic or acute, and were on dialysis three days a week. Their quality of life was severely compromised. It's an arduous process to be evaluated and approved to go on the transplant list, and most patients on the list will never receive a kidney because of the shortage of donors, both living and deceased. Again, part of my responsibility was to offer hope that they would not be forgotten while they were waiting, and remind them there was the possibility of a transplant any day, so it was critical they maintain their health in the most positive way they could and stay in communication with the transplant team.

This involved not only the patient but also the family. It was very rewarding and humbling to be in the operating room when the patient received the new kidney and see it pink up and begin to produce urine as soon as it was connected. Of course, after the transplant, new challenges were there for the patient—antirejection medications and endless follow-up visits with the doctors. Still, we offered patients hope that they could manage these new demands and that we would guide them through the process and be there for them.

Two years later, I made another change. I became a cancer research nurse. This may sound like a boring or even depressing job, but it was actually very uplifting, inspiring, challenging, and rewarding. I was primarily responsible for phase 1 clinical trials, which usually involved first-in-human drugs. The patients considered for these types of trials had advanced disease and had usually exhausted all standard-of-care treatments and had no other options available to them. They knew their chances for a cure were minimal, but they also knew we would do everything possible so they received the best possible treatment available; they wouldn't suffer; and they would still have a sense of autonomy and some control over their bodies and their decisions. We offered compassionate honesty and treated them with respect. My job was to guide patients through the trial and be their voice and advocate as well as a professional and ethical researcher for the pharmaceutical companies sponsoring the trials and the institution conducting the trials.

Part of my responsibility was to carefully explain the purpose of the trial, the screening process to ensure eligibility to go on the trial, what would be expected of patients while they were on the trial, and, most difficult, that there was no guarantee the new drug would work for them. I did this in a way that still offered honest hope. I told them I would be their "new best friend" through it all. I told them they would have my direct office number and they should call if they had questions, problems, or were experiencing anything that didn't seem right. I told them we would do everything we could to make the trial procedures and treatments as tolerable as possible and that they would always have the choice to discontinue treatment and go off the trial at any time if that was their desire. Their family was also an important part of this process.

The consent to go on a clinical trial can be twenty, thirty, or forty pages long, filled with scary possible side effects, unfamiliar words, required tests, and a schedule that seems overwhelming to manage. It is up to the oncologist and the research nurse to explain the consent in a way the patient and the family can understand, so they are giving an informed consent and know why they're being offered a clinical trial at this particular time. Some patients wanted to sign it right away without reading it. That is not being informed. At this time, they still felt overwhelmed by the news they had just received that their disease had progressed and there were no other treatments available.

I encouraged my patients to take the consent home, read through it with their family, make notes, write down questions, and then return the next day so we could discuss it in a way that they understood the consent and felt comfortable signing it. If they lived out of town, I found a quiet place where they could read through it together. When they returned, I always started with the patient and family, asking them to tell me what they understood about the consent and the trial, and to voice their questions and concerns honestly and openly. I wanted to know what they understood and where they were at emotionally. Then we went through the consent together. I had an ethical responsibility to be sure they understood the risks and possible benefits of the trial, and I never took that lightly.

In all these different positions, the common thread was the possibility of hope—for survival, for dignity, for pain management, for compassion, for empathy, for integrity, for connection, to be seen and heard, for autonomy. Especially as a cancer research nurse, I believe this sincere sense of hope offered them truth, peace, courage, strength, faith, and love. I was also a safe place for them to share their grief, fears, tears, and anger. For me, I was able to share with them my own experiences, my passion, my values, and my love in a way that had never been possible or available for me before. I was blessed to be at the perfect place at the perfect time in my life.

Hope takes many forms. Working with all these beautiful, courageous people, having all these challenging experiences, taught me how to live my own life with hope, faith, compassion, courage, and integrity at a deeper level than I ever imagined. It is my sincere hope to share with you what I have learned from these teachers so you may find your own source of hope and be empowered to create a life you love through the gift of hope and love, even in the darkness of fear and grief.

I retired as a research nurse after almost ten years. It was the most profound experience I ever had. I will always be grateful.

> *You're worried about how you're going to feel at the end of your life? What about right now? Live. Right in this minute. That's where the joy's at.*
> *—Abigail Thomas, author, memoirist*

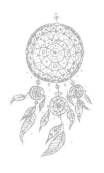

CHAPTER 1

MYTHS

Look deeper into the actions you take and the truths you take for granted. Ask why and then ask why again.
—*Walter Mosley, American novelist*

There are several myths, pieces of misinformation, and stigmas surrounding cancer. Some sound ridiculous now, others are still believed, and some may actually have a grain of truth.

I remember as a child, no one ever said the C-word. It was as if it was a deep dark secret or a profanity that wasn't spoken in polite company. At the same time, there was a belief that cancer was contagious, so the patient was isolated from family, friends, and coworkers (if they were able to still work). Surgery wasn't considered an option because of the belief that the air would spread the cancer if the patient was "opened up."

Most people thought then, and to some extent even now, that cancer was always terminal or that the treatment was worse than the disease. So imagine not being able to talk about your disease with anyone, being isolated from everyone, not having a treatment option, and believing you're going to die any day, suffer from horrendous side effects, and be in pain until that final day comes.

Other common myths are *I have no family history of cancer, I'm too young or I'm too old to get cancer, I've never smoked, I eat a healthy diet.* There are still many myths and inaccuracies surrounding cancer that cause patients to feel isolated, guilty, ashamed, pitied, fearful, powerless, or in denial.

BLAME MYTHS

If a patient has cancer, it must be their fault in some way.

Everything happens for a reason.

You can win the battle against cancer if you're mentally strong enough, have willpower and the right attitude.

Some patients believe if they had just been stronger, prayed more, meditated more, visualized more, manifested more, they would have been the victor. So when these measures fail and the cancer worsens or progresses, they feel like they're to blame.

EMPOWERMENT TRUTHS

I believe a good attitude is important in dealing with any health crisis, or life crisis for that matter. Although a positive attitude is important for overall well-being, by itself it's not enough and causes people to feel guilty if they don't respond. It's been my observation, however, that people with a positive outlook tended to manage their cancer diagnosis and treatments better, and their quality of life was certainly better.

Cancer is not a battle of good over evil, right over wrong, strength over weakness. Cancer's not personal. Cancer doesn't care.

A good attitude, affirmations, positive visualizations, and mantras by themselves are not enough. You cannot *will* cancer away. You cannot *pray* cancer away, although faith is very important—faith in yourself, faith in your health care team, and faith in your individual spiritual or religious beliefs. Prayers offer peace and hope, but they're to be used along with treatment, not instead of it. There are supportive measures that are of benefit, like meditation, mindfulness, healthy eating, and exercise. These not only improve your overall sense of well-being but help support your immune system.

Pray, meditate, or do whatever brings you relief, because these things help you to cope and give you a respite from the exhaustion of cancer that on some days may seem overwhelming. Do these things to help support your immune system and your mental, emotional, and spiritual needs. Discover what works for you—a nap, a walk in nature, music, a good book, socializing with friends. This is about you, no one else. It's about your quality of life and what's important to you. Quality of life is always the bottom line.

Do not allow yourself to become isolated, unseen and unheard.

COMMUNITY AND INTERNET MYTHS

Don't tell anyone you have cancer, because you might lose your job, your friends, or you'll become a burden to your family, or people will pity you, shun you.

This Internet product or person will "cure" your cancer.

Be careful who you talk to and listen to about your cancer diagnosis, treatments, life expectancy, cures. Don't super-surf the Internet. There are reliable resources like the American Cancer Society and the National Cancer Institute that offer proven, reliable information. There's a lot of false or misleading information on the Internet that will drive you crazy, increase your anxiety, and make you question everything that's happening to you—or cause you to spend your life savings on a product or person with unproven "cures."

COMMUNICATION TRUTHS

Every cancer is a little different, and everyone experiences it and responds a little differently. What one person experiences may not be what you experience. Well-intentioned people may want to talk to you about their own experience or the experiences of others they've known with cancer. Listen with an open, but cautious, mind.

One patient had sarcoma that had spread to his lungs. He told his friends, and they thought he had lung cancer. They were giving him all kinds of advice about lung cancer even though they had no personal experience.

His cancer was not lung cancer. It was a totally different type of cancer and required a different type of treatment. He came to the clinic confused and worried. We explained to him the difference between a sarcoma that had metastasized to his lungs and primary lung cancer—two very different diseases.

While it's important for others to share information and offer support, make sure the information you're receiving is correct and of positive value to you. Always talk with your healthcare provider about any questions or concerns you may have. You're not exactly like anyone else, and the way you respond to treatment may not be the same as someone else. Your oncology team has heard these same questions, concerns, and myths during their careers and can share the latest scientific data so you can make educated, informed decisions about your care that are right for you.

AGE MYTHS

Cancer, excluding childhood cancers, only occurs in older people.

If my child gets the HPV (human papilloma virus) vaccine, they'll be encouraged to become sexually active.

My child is too young to talk about sex or "sexual" cancers.

AGE TRUTHS

Younger people are developing certain cancers at a higher rate. Studies have shown an increase in certain cancers in people under fifty and even under twenty-five.

Colon cancer is now being diagnosed in younger people, some under the age of forty-five, especially people of color. People in this population are often underserved, have limited access to screening, feel embarrassed, have culture-based ideas about cancer or screening procedures, or are in denial that they could be at risk. Many insurance companies are now recommending colonoscopies for people age forty-five and older. Colon cancer is not an old-age cancer.

Certain HPV-related cancers, such as cervical cancer and some oral and anal cancers, are caused by the HPV virus, so they could possibly be considered contagious. That's why the HPV vaccine for boys, girls, men, and women ages eleven to forty-six is so important. Recently, there was a documented report of a woman developing a rare HPV squamous-cell skin cancer after her cuticle was cut, possibly due to unclean equipment.

According to a *Guardian* article published on August 22, 2022, Rwanda is on track to become the first country to wipe out cervical cancer, the most common cancer in that country and fourth most common cancer in women worldwide. The Rwandan government is doing this through a very proactive and aggressive campaign to provide community screenings for all women and HPV vaccines for twelve-year-old girls in school, plus early treatment for those found to be precancerous.

Rwanda has demonstrated the importance of women in their community. They support the empowerment and wellness of women and are not connecting cancer with sex or as something taboo or shameful. Such measures could/should be possible in this country.

Risk factors for certain cancers may be childhood obesity, high fat diet, consumption of sugary drinks, lack of physical activity, smoking, vaping, adolescent binge drinking, and use of birth-control pills. One positive factor in the increase of certain cancers may be early detection through screening and diagnosing cancers at an earlier stage than was previously possible.

LUNG CANCER MYTHS

Only smokers get lung cancer.

Vaping doesn't cause lung cancer.

I won't get lung cancer if I don't inhale.

If I quit smoking after having smoked for a long time, I'll actually get lung cancer because my body misses the tobacco.

LUNG CANCER TRUTHS

According to the American Cancer Society, in 2020 about 12 percent of lung cancers were in patients who never smoked. Lung cancer can be caused by secondhand smoke, radon, and environmental factors, such as air pollution, or from an unknown cause. Recently, researchers at the National Cancer Institute and other sites have used whole-genome sequencing to characterize three molecular subtypes of lung cancer in people who had never smoked. In addition, some people who have smoked most of their lives have, by sheer luck or fate, never gotten lung cancer, which in some ways doesn't seem fair. But they may have contracted other cancers, such as oral cancers, esophageal cancer, or certain lymphomas. Of course, smokers are also at risk for other diseases, such as heart disease and strokes. There are no benefits to smoking.

My mother died of lymphoma at the age of seventy-nine, two months shy of her eightieth birthday. She had smoked heavily since the age of fourteen. It was the cool thing for women to do during and after World War II. She was addicted to smoking. She had no desire to quit. She would walk through a snowstorm to the corner store if she thought she was going to run out of cigarettes. She smoked her last cigarette as the EMTs were taking her down the steps on a stretcher and into the ambulance for her trip to hospice, where she died the next day.

Smoking is addictive and scientifically, clinically proven to be linked to increases in lung cancer as well as other diseases, such as heart disease. This may be especially true for younger people who are now vaping. They may have precancerous disease or compromised cardiovascular function that will show itself later in adulthood. Many cases of lung cancer may have been and could have been prevented by not smoking or using any kind of tobacco product. Cancer is opportunistic, and smoking, vaping, or chewing tobacco opens the door for cancer to walk through and settle in.

BREAST CANCER MYTHS

Men don't get breast cancer.
  I don't have a family history of breast cancer.
  I'm too young to have breast cancer.

BREAST CANCER TRUTHS

About 1 percent of breast cancers occur in men. Although a small number, the mortality rate is high because of the delay in diagnosis and treatment due to embarrassment, denial, and lack of resources for male mammograms.

Most breast cancers occur in women, and men, with no family history of breast cancer. You may not have a reliable, clear history of a family member's cancer, such as the presence of a BRCA gene mutation. Women, especially women of color, are developing breast cancer at a younger age, particularly triple negative breast cancer, the most aggressive form. Unfortunately, they're often not diagnosed until the disease has advanced because they don't have convenient access, or they don't have insurance, are underinsured, or the insurance company won't pay for a mammogram or an ultrasound because of their younger age. When the cancer is diagnosed at an advanced stage due to delays in screening, the cancer is more difficult to treat, and the prognosis may be poorer.

Sometimes a lump is dismissed as "nothing" because of the woman's young age. Don't take no for an answer. Get a second opinion, or a third. It's your body and your future. Learn how to do monthly breast self-exams. Know the early warning signs of breast cancer, and schedule an annual mammogram or ultrasound if appropriate.

I remember in 1976, when I was a second-year nursing student on my surgical/OR rotation, a patient who had an undiagnosed lump in her breast was scheduled for surgery. A biopsy of the lump had not been taken. The consent she signed stated she would have a radical mastectomy if the lump was malignant. That meant she would be waking up from anesthesia not knowing if she still had a breast. That was considered standard-of-care at the time, at least at the hospital where I worked.

Thankfully, that's no longer the case. Women can have a lumpectomy and then, based on the diagnosis and the recommendations of her breast surgeon and oncologist, make the decision as to what is the best course of treatment for her—further surgery, radiation therapy, chemotherapy, or a combination of treatments. Patients should always have power over their own body.

SURGERY MYTHS

Surgery causes the cancer to spread when the air hits it.

If the surgeon sees cancer, he'll just close me up because there's nothing that can be done.

SURGERY TRUTHS

Exposure to air doesn't spread cancer during surgery. Sometimes more extensive cancer is discovered during surgery because it didn't originally appear on the scans but was still there. The surgeon is anticipating what may be discovered during surgery and has a plan of action.

Many cancers are successfully treated with surgical intervention, sometimes in conjunction with other treatment modalities, such as chemotherapy and/or radiation. Your cancer surgeon will explain the risks and benefits of surgery, possible options, and what the proper course is for your particular cancer.

You are an active partner in these decisions, not a sideliner. Ask questions and keep asking until you comfortably understand the procedure, risks, and benefits. Your questions, your concerns, and your fears should be treated with honesty and respect.

TREATMENT MYTHS

Treatment is worse than the disease.

Holistic medicine is a natural cure.

I remember going to a cancer hospital on business in the late seventies or early eighties. It looked like a prison from the outside—tall, almost windowless, with grey concrete walls. Inside, the walls were sterile white. It was deathly quiet. There was a medicinal odor that lingered—perhaps cleaning chemicals used to sanitize the vomiting and incontinence from the patients. Or perhaps the smell was the chemotherapy drugs being administered in almost lethal doses and combinations at the time.

Patients were kept behind closed doors and isolated from one another. Their only visitors were the nurses tending to them and occasionally the oncologist. Back then, the treatment *was* worse than the disease.

A current popular myth is that holistic and naturopathic medicines are natural cures for cancer. A patient came to talk to us about a clinical trial for metastatic (stage 4) melanoma. He had recently been diagnosed and was referred to us by his primary physician. He was in his forties, working full time, physically active, and otherwise healthy—a perfect candidate for this clinical trial.

We explained the trial and the success patients were having with this new immunotherapy drug. We explained that this drug would bolster his own immune system to attack the melanoma cells, and any side effects he might experience would be carefully monitored and effectively managed. He listened and said he would think about it. We explained that he didn't have the luxury of time, as the melanoma was aggressive and, if left untreated, would quickly spread and worsen.

He then told us that his daughter was a *curandera*, a healer, who had trained in Mexico. She told him she could "cure" him with "natural" treatments and "healing" ceremonies, and he should not take any "toxic" pharmaceuticals. We tried to explain to him that we could talk with his daughter and explain what we were doing and how her approach could be incorporated with accepted and proven treatment. He declined.

He died shortly thereafter, with the melanoma having spread to his brain. His belief in his daughter outweighed his belief in the science of the treatment. He thought he had to choose between the two.

TREATMENT TRUTHS

Cancer centers today are modern, with a positive and upbeat attitude. Patients can share their experiences with one another and offer support to one another. Family members and loved ones are encouraged to visit (except during COVID). The staff is hopeful and energetic and professional. It is a feeling of family, support, hope, and trust.

Holistic medicine can be used in conjunction with standard cancer therapies if approved by your oncologist. However, some herbs, fruits, vegetables, and over-the-counter medications such as vitamins and supplements can actually interfere with the effectiveness of some treatments. Tell your oncologist about any herbs, supplements, and medications, both prescribed and over-the-counter, you're taking.

The Native American population was encouraged to meet with their Medicine Man for additional support if that was their wish, but any treatments or ceremonies were to be discussed with the oncologist first to be sure they were safe for the patient. Cultural beliefs, if appropriate, were supported.

SIDE EFFECT MYTHS

Side effects from the treatments will be worse than the disease, so I'd rather do nothing and let nature take its course.

I don't want to get treatment because I'm afraid I'll lose my hair.

I'm afraid I'll be in bed all the time because I'll be too weak to do the things I enjoy.

I'm afraid I won't be able to eat the foods I enjoy because of overwhelming and uncontrollable nausea and vomiting or diarrhea.

SIDE EFFECT TRUTHS

Today, side effects like pain, nausea, vomiting, diarrhea, and anemia can be successfully treated and managed with medications and other treatment options, such as palliative care. However, you do have to communicate with your health care provider that you're having these side effects. There is no need to suffer in silence. As I used to tell my patients, you don't get extra points for suffering. Suffering in silence is not about bravery or being strong.

Some patients are afraid or reluctant to tell their oncologist about the side effects they're experiencing because they think they'll have to come off treatment, especially if they're on a clinical trial with no other available treatment options. It's better to tell someone than try to hide any side effects that may be causing you more harm and may lead to hospitalization when they could have been managed effectively when they first appeared.

HOSPICE MYTHS

Hospice is a last resort that means everyone has given up and the patient is just left to die alone.

HOSPICE/PALLIATIVE CARE TRUTHS

Hospice and palliative care may be a difficult choice for family members or loved ones to accept, but it's far from a dumping ground for the patient. It is a way for a patient with no further treatment options or who has chosen not to receive any further treatment to get supportive care by professionals trained and experienced in delivering this specialized care and support. Hospice can be outpatient at the patient's home or inpatient in a specialized setting in a hospital or center, depending on the needs and wishes of the patient and the family.

Hospice includes pain management with medication, and emotional support, including social worker support, clerical support if requested, and support in diminishing any side effects, such as nausea, vomiting, or diarrhea. Support also includes physical care, such as bathing, turning in bed, assisted walking if possible, and dietary support. Inpatient hospice is not a nursing home. It is a place of safety, the highest standard of care, and a place where the family is supported, welcomed, and encouraged to be with their loved one. Outpatient hospice offers support not only to the patient but also to the family caring for the patient.

CLINICAL TRIAL MYTHS

There's a cure for cancer but the doctors and pharmaceutical companies are hiding it.
You're a guinea pig if you go on a clinical trial.
Clinical trials use placebos, not real medicine.

CLINICAL TRIAL TRUTHS

Cancer is not a single disease. There is not one cure. It is hundreds of diseases that respond differently to different treatments and in different patients. Clinical trials are the future for more effective, more tolerable cancer treatments and supportive care. Without trials, we wouldn't have any of the new drugs we have today, which have been proven to be effective. We wouldn't have new surgical techniques and radiation therapy treatments.

People who enroll in a clinical trial are not thought of as guinea pigs. Most are going on the trial because they hope the treatment will be effective for them. Many are also doing it for altruistic reasons—hoping a new drug will be discovered that will treat future patients like them in a more effective, lifesaving way. People enrolled in clinical trials are heroes. They are selfless. They have courageous optimism.

There are four phases of clinical trials:

- **Phase 1** is usually a first-in-human drug or a drug that has been used for another purpose, such as treating a different type of cancer. A limited number of patients are enrolled in a phase 1 trial that usually involves only a few cancer centers and a small number of patients. The endpoint of the trial is to determine the side effects (mild to serious) and the maximum tolerated dose for the drug.
- After the phase 1 data is submitted and carefully reviewed by peers and the FDA and deemed to be safe and efficacious, the benefits outweighing the risks, the trial enters **phase 2** with more patients and more centers enrolled.
- Data is once again submitted and reviewed by the FDA and, if deemed appropriate, becomes a **phase 3** trial.

This process can take years. Sometimes a drug is so promising and side effects so manageable, with the benefits markedly outweighing the risks, that a drug becomes available sooner (fast-tracked) so patients who have no other treatment options can receive promising care in the timeliest manner. This is what happened with the early immunotherapy drugs in clinical trials for melanoma.

I was fortunate to be a part of those early trials, and the results were amazing. No, not everyone was cured, and some had very serious side effects that were diligently treated, but many experienced at least a partial response, which was promising when there had been no other treatment options available offering the same results. They were given more time with an acceptable quality of life, which was the most precious thing for them. Now, five years after I retired, new patients receiving these drugs are showing no evidence of disease and living a good quality of life.

According to the American Cancer Society, in 2022, an estimated 1.9 million new cancer cases will be diagnosed, and 609,360 people will die of cancer diseases. The Biden "moonshot initiative" hopes to decrease US cancer fatalities by 50 percent over the next twenty-five years. In my opinion, this is too long and too politically driven. How many more of these deaths could be prevented by readily available preventive measures, like more aggressive awareness and education of cancer risks, earlier screening for all populations, and better availability of clinical trials for patients? Now is the time to be proactive in education, screening, and diagnosing cancers, and making cancer treatments and trials more available to more patients.

THE GOOD NEWS

According to the National Cancer Institute's Office of Cancer Survivorship, the number of people with a history of cancer in the

United States has increased dramatically, from 3 million in 1971 to about 14.5 million today. About 64 percent of today's cancer survivors were diagnosed with cancer five or more years ago. Approximately 15 percent of all cancer survivors were diagnosed twenty or more years ago. Over the next decade, the number of people who have lived five years or more after a cancer diagnosis is expected to increase by approximately 37 percent.

This is real hope, not fantasy. It's not just about surviving cancer, but quality of life. More patients today are living with cancer and enjoying a good quality of life. They've become active partners in their cancer management and have found a way for cancer to not be seen as a ruthless enemy.

I have been seeing more commercials on TV promoting new cancer therapies. What I like about them, in addition to being informative, is that they show normal people living normal lives. This is the future for cancer treatments and cancer patients.

Cancer is a team disease. It requires patients, oncologists, surgeons, radiation oncologists, chemotherapy/infusion nurses, research nurses, patient nurse navigators, social workers, geneticists, pharmacists, scientists, and many others who show up every day committed to doing their best to make a positive difference for patients they may or may not ever see. Many of these people work behind the scenes, but they are all equally important as more strides, more discoveries are made in the unraveling and unveiling of this disease.

I have never worked with a team of health care professionals who worked every day with so much hope, determination, commitment, high ethical standards, compassion, empathy, and integrity. I've never worked with patients who showed so much courage, faith, trust, and hope. It was an experience that changed me in so many ways, and I'll always be grateful.

*Taking responsibility for your beliefs and judgments gives
you the power to change them.*
                                    —*Byron Katie, American speaker and author,*
                                                      creator of The Work.

JOURNAL

- What myths, misinformation, denials about cancer are you holding on to, keeping each one alive, feeding it by defending it so it keeps growing stronger?
- How are you justifying this holding on? How can you Iet go?
- Do you identify yourself as a cancer patient or as a human being who happens to have cancer? The first leaves you feeling like a victim. The second gives you strength and hope.
- What if you could step back for even a moment and ask yourself, *Is this really true? Is this my truth now? Does holding on to this belief and this pain support me or allow me to be who I truly am?*
- What would be possible for you if you acknowledged new truths and released the old ways of thinking?
- Do you believe that prevention and the development of new advanced treatments could significantly impact the incidence and the death rate of cancer in the foreseeable future?
- Are you an advocate and supporter for continued cancer research? Everyone can do something, whether it's contributing to one of the many cancer research organizations, improving education about cancer, promoting earlier and more accessible cancer screening in your community, volunteering at your local cancer center, or, if a patient, enrolling in a clinical trial if appropriate. This is a worldwide disease that effects millions of people, and we each have something positive we can contribute to changing its course.

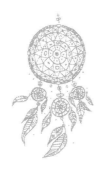

CHAPTER 2

GRIEF

The reality is that you will grieve forever. You will not "get over" the loss of a loved one; you will learn to live with it. You will heal and you will rebuild yourself around the loss you have suffered. You will be whole again but you will never be the same. Nor should you be the same nor would you want to.

—Elisabeth Kübler-Ross, psychiatrist,
author of On Death and Dying

What is grief? According to the New Oxford American Dictionary, grief is "deep sorrow, especially that caused by someone's death." For me, that is a very superficial interpretation of grief. Grief is felt and experienced differently by everyone. There is no recipe for how to handle it.

Grief isn't just about the loss of a loved one. Grief is the real or perceived loss of anything that is sacred and precious in our lives, including our own self. We grieve the person we thought we were. We grieve the person we thought we'd be. Grief is the expression of loss of any kind—a person, a beloved pet, a lover, a friend, an idea or belief taken away.

Grief is the loss of a job, resulting in the loss of our own self-worth and ability to provide and care for ourselves and others. Grief is financial loss resulting in bankruptcy and the loss of our identity as a responsible, successful person. We can experience grief as a change in our body image, such as the loss of hair that had been our crown; the inability to enjoy a meal we once looked forward to; loss of weight resulting in fatigue and inability to enjoy the things we loved or to care for ourselves; loss of a body part and our own self-image and self-identify. Grief is multifaceted and multilayered.

Grief manifests in many forms—denial, anger, resentment, isolation, fear, guilt, blame, disappointment, manipulation. Grief is a chameleon seemingly blending into everything surrounding us. There is no timetable for grief. There is no one solution to overcoming grief. Grief becomes the master of our soul, our heart. Grief leaves on its own schedule or may shackle itself to us forever. Grief is complicated to accept and understand.

We're told to be strong. We're told everything will be better. We're told we don't have it as bad as some other people in the same situation. We're told we're supposed to cry and mourn in silence, in privacy, so as not to make others feel uncomfortable or pity us. We're told we shouldn't feel at peace or worse, be happy or laugh ever again. *Lies!*

Health care professionals also experience grief. It may be the sadness following the loss of a patient they had tried so hard to treat and had come to know as more than just a patient. It may be a sense of personal failure—if they had just done a little more, knowing no more could have been done. If the patient had just come to them a little sooner. Grief is swallowed and pushed down into the deepest part of themselves so they can move on to the next patient who needs the professionals to be totally present. Grief is a luxury they can't afford.

No one is immune to grief. There is no vaccine for grief. Grief wakes you up in the middle of the night asking yourself how you will go on, how much more can you give, how much more do you have to give. Can love, empathy, compassion, and grief in all its forms coexist?

Grief isn't one emotion. It may even be the absence of emotion. A heart frozen. A mind numbed. Grief appears in many forms, and each one is real, each one a path through darkness with no one to guide you.

> *Words can never say what we truly want them to say, for they fumble, stammer and break the best porcelain. The best one can hope for is to find along the way someone to share the path, content to walk in silence, for the heart communes best when it does not try to speak.*
>
> —*Margaret Weis, American fantasy*
> *and science fiction writer who has sold*
> *more than 30 million books internationally*

GRIEF IS A JOURNEY TAKEN ALONE

I have felt guilty and wondered if there was something wrong with me for not grieving for my mom when she passed, at least not in the "normal, accepted, correct, traditional" way. We'd had a complicated relationship throughout my life. My mom died of lymphoma at the age of seventy-nine, just two months before she turned eighty. I was fifty-seven, newly divorced, and had just re-entered nursing as a kidney-transplant coordinator.

We lived in different states, and I went to visit periodically, especially on Mother's Day—my mom's favorite holiday. We talked on the phone, but these were usually short conversations without much substance. Some days, she wouldn't answer the phone when I called, causing me to wonder if she was OK. I had been worried about my mom for some time because she lived alone, and I always had the fear I would get a phone call saying she had been found dead in her apartment.

One day, she told me she hadn't been feeling well, had actually been in the hospital for a few days, but it was "nothing" and not to worry. A few months after her hospitalization, I got a call from a doctor telling me he was my mom's oncologist and had been treating her for lymphoma. I was speechless and wasn't sure I was hearing him correctly. I really didn't understand the depth of that diagnosis at the time. Since she was a smoker, I would have been less surprised if he had said she had lung cancer. But lymphoma? How? Why?

He said I should come see her. I told him I would try to get some time off from work and would be there in a few weeks. He said, "No, you have to come now." He said my mom had told him she was done with treatment and asked him how long she would live without further treatment. He told her it could be four weeks to six months. She told him she would take four weeks. I went to see her right away, not knowing what to expect and still unable to process this news.

She told me what had been happening with her, and she was at peace with it. She was choosing to live for four weeks and would like to live those weeks with me. I think she felt she would be safe with me, and I would respect her wishes. Of course I said yes.

My mom had very few possessions, and what she had, she had already given away. The rest was sent to me in a couple of cardboard boxes. She found a good home for her sweet dog, Sophie, even though I told her she could come with us.

When we got to my apartment, I arranged for in-home hospice care. She had told me she wanted to be cremated. I ordered the urn on eBay.

It was called Purple Passion, which I thought was very appropriate for her, since purple was her favorite color and she had led a very passionate life (married seven or eight times, but who's counting).

For the first three weeks she lived with me, she was actually feeling pretty well. She was eating, laughing, and even doing some shopping (her favorite hobby). I thought, hoped, maybe she was recovering—I didn't understand how silently lymphoma progresses. I think she had allowed herself to relax because she finally felt safe being with me.

The fourth week, she started rapidly declining. I would lie in bed at night listening for her breathing. Even though I was a nurse, every time I gave her the pain pills given to me by the hospice nurse, I was scared I might accidentally overdose her. Being a nurse for a patient is very different from being the daughter of a patient.

Finally, on the Friday of the fourth week, I called the hospice nurse and told her I thought it was time for inpatient hospice so she would be better cared for 24–7. The nurse came, assessed her, and agreed. The next day, Saturday morning, I got the call that I had better come to the facility, because she wasn't expected to live much longer.

I waited. A few hours later, the call came that she had passed, exactly four weeks to the day of her decision. My mom had told me she didn't want anyone to be there with her when she died. I don't know why.

While she was living with me, we talked a lot about our past experiences and differences. We laughed about the funny things, said we were sorry for the unhappy things. She told me how much she loved me and how proud she was of me. I told her I loved her, and because of her, I had become the person I was—independent, caring, and forgiving. But we didn't talk about those last moments, what it would be like for her and for me. She knew I would respect her wishes, even though it was painful for me.

I took comfort in knowing a caregiver was with her, holding her hand, when she passed. I waited a few hours before I went to get her things. Upon arrival, I wasn't prepared for what I saw—the gurney carrying her sheet-wrapped body out to the hearse. I wished I had waited a little longer. That was not the last memory I expected or wanted to have of her.

I met with the hospice charge nurse, picked up a brown paper bag with her few things, and told the nurse I had to leave and be somewhere where people were alive and living their lives. At that moment, I couldn't be around death and dying. She looked at me in a puzzled way and probably thought I was a very callous and ungrateful daughter, but it was because I had cared so much, loved so deeply, that I had to find some source of life to hold me up at that moment. I had given her a safe space for her final weeks; she was not in pain or suffering. I just needed at that moment to be around living, creative people and see that life goes on and it's beautiful. She would have wanted that.

It's not that I didn't care, but I was going to grieve in my own way, not a prescribed script about how I should grieve. I went to an outdoor art festival and let the creative, happy energy permeate me and fill my soul. I allowed myself to breathe deeply and let go.

The hospice caregiver told me that my mother's last words were, "I'm done, I'm ready to go home now." Those were the words she always said when she was ready to leave the bar after a night of dancing. Those words give me peace knowing she left her way, on her terms, and she wasn't suffering. It was just one more dance.

> *Your legs will get heavy and tired. Then comes a moment of feeling the wings you've grown, lifting.*
> —*Rumi: Selected Poems*

A week after she died, I picked up the urn with her ashes. It wasn't very heavy. It was difficult to comprehend that her whole life, her whole being, was in that container. It was her ashes but not her. I held it to my chest, but there was no warmth, no hug returned. Could she feel me? Could she hear the words I said to her as I took her home?

When I returned to work that Monday, the social worker in the transplant department told me I wasn't handling my grief "properly" because I had returned to work so soon and wasn't crying. She told me I must be in denial. She had no idea what I was feeling on the inside, what my mom and I had been through together all those years and in those final days, all the tears that had been shed through our lifetimes. There was nothing else for me to do for her or for me.

> Sometimes tears have risen miles before they brim in the eyes.
>
> —James Richardson

No one has the right to tell you how to grieve. Grief is the most personal emotion someone can experience. There is no "healthy" way to grieve. I miss my mom every day, and there are days when I wonder if I made the right decision to not be there when she passed, as she had requested. There are days and nighttime dreams when I feel and see her presence next to me.

A few days after she passed, I went through her address book to see if there was anybody I should notify of her passing. I put it back in my desk drawer. A few months later, for whatever reason, I took it out again. This time I saw on the inside cover her handwritten words: *courage, faith, truth, love*. I had looked at this page several times before, but this was the first time I saw those words. I believe this was my mom's message to me about how to live my life, because in the end, that's all there is. I had this cover page cut out and framed so I see it every day and remind myself what's important in my life.

> *There's freedom in knowing you can carry joy and grief together.*
>
> —*Nancy Berns, author, speaker,*
> *and professor of sociology*

GRIEF BURROWS INTO THE HEART

I came to understand grief on a deeper level after I became a cancer research nurse and worked so closely with patients and their families. Everyone experienced grief differently. Everyone was on a different part of their own path. Some were mired in their grief, and some traveled gracefully and bravely through it, or so it seemed to an outsider. Some were in denial and refused to talk about what was happening or might happen, as if talking about it would make it happen sooner, make it too real.

Each person we met had to be supported and respected for where they were and be gently guided to a more comforting and positive place if possible. Some patients or their family members lashed out at us verbally and sometimes even physically because they were so scared and their pain was so great. This could not be tolerated and had to be dealt with in a professional, gentle manner, even if we sometimes wanted to lash back and tell them we were there to help them, we were on their side, we didn't cause this to happen to them, it wasn't our fault. We also had feelings for them and their loved ones. We were dealing with our own grief for them.

One patient had been an air traffic controller for over thirty years. He kept working long past his eligibility for retirement, saying they were short-staffed, no one else had his experience, no one else could do the job as well as he could. Shortly after he finally retired, he started having a cough that wouldn't go away. He finally went to his family doctor, a chest X-ray was taken, and a mass was seen. A CT scan was done, and he was diagnosed with stage 4 lung cancer.

He was so angry. He said, "I've worked my whole life, I've never smoked or drank, I ate the right foods and exercised every day. How could I have lung cancer? It's not fair. Why me?" We tried to explain to him that it was not his fault.

After going through standard-of-care treatments for his type of lung cancer (a genetic mutation not related to smoking), he chose to go on a phase 1 clinical trial using targeted therapy specific to his type of lung cancer. He tolerated the trial well, but each time he came to the clinic, I could sense his anger and resentment for having to spend his day at this place, be around other cancer patients, and go through the treatments. All of these surroundings reminded him of his disease and the uncertainty of life after he had spent a lifetime planning every moment, always in control, professionally and personally.

Unfortunately he didn't respond to the treatment, although other patients on the same trial did. The drug went on to be cleared by the FDA and is now part of a standard-of-care treatment regimen. I wonder how much his negative mental attitude, anger, hopelessness, and grief played in his outcome. His wife tried to be supportive, but she was dealing with her own grief and the loss she knew she would soon be facing—her life partner of so many years.

For me as a nurse, one of the hardest things was seeing patients who had worked through their own grief and had found a place of peace and acceptance while a family member or loved one was still in the storm of grief, feeling drowned by it, unable to find a place of resolution or reason.

The patient tried to comfort the family, but the family wasn't ready to let go, to accept the inevitable, so everyone suffered.

Grief can eventually bring closure. It can also bring anger, resentment, and divisiveness that may go unaddressed and untreated until it's too late. Grief can bring up old wounds, old hurts that had been lying dormant or festering for years. These can't be treated with cancer drugs.

Another patient was in a different part of her cancer journey. She had been through all the standard-of-care treatments and chose to go on a phase 1 trial in the hope this would be the "cure" or at least help someone else in the future. Unfortunately, her disease continued to progress. She accepted that there were no other treatments available for her. Her only request was that her pain would be managed effectively.

However, her adult sons were still dealing with their own grief. One was very angry that there was nothing more that could be done for his mother. He couldn't believe she had no other treatment options. The other was beginning to understand the reality of the situation, although not quite at the point of accepting it. When they came to the clinic with their mother, they started arguing as soon as they entered the cancer center and continued it in the exam room, where their mother was waiting to be seen. The argument became quite heated. The mother just sat there, not crying, not talking, shrinking into herself, maybe wishing it was already over.

When I came into the room and heard the arguing, I asked the men to leave and wait in the waiting room. I then talked to their mom and asked her how she was feeling about what happened. She said it happened all the time at home, and she just couldn't deal with it anymore. She didn't know how to talk to them, how to tell them how she was feeling, what her final wishes were. She couldn't tell them that she loved them because they told her if she loved them she would keep fighting to live for them.

They weren't bad sons. They just couldn't get past their anger and their fears to give her the comfort and support she desperately needed. She was referred to palliative care for management of her pain and to receive comfort care for her physical and emotional needs. The sons were left with their grief.

I wish we had had grief counselors available for patients and their families. Would that have made their journeys any easier? I would like to see every cancer center have grief counselors on staff—it could make such a difference for everyone—patients, family, caregivers, professional staff.

GRIEF AS FEAR AND GUILT

Once you face your fear, nothing is ever as hard as you think.

—Olivia Newton-John, singer, actress

Fear and guilt are overwhelming. They are real. They are unspeakable.

The survivor says, *You tell me I have nothing to worry about, I'll get through this. But there's so much you don't know. I'm not that strong. He/she was the strong one, the smart one, the planner, the one who took care of everything. He/she took care of me. How do I take care of myself at this point in my life? I don't want to appear needy. I don't want to ask for help. I don't want pity. I should be able to do this by myself. I never thought it would end this way. I thought he/she would be the one to go first. I never thought of it at all.*

Who will take care of me? How will I survive by myself? Can I afford to keep the house we've had all these years? How can I leave this home we shared and all the memories it holds? How can I live looking at these memories every day? Who will host the Thanksgiving, Christmas, Easter, birthday, anniversary dinners? How do I cook for one? How can I go out to eat by myself? How can I travel by myself?

Am I betraying the one I loved if I feel happy, if I plan a trip, if I meet with friends, if I sell the house? Will there still be friends we knew as a couple now that I'm alone? What about the finances? Was there an insurance policy? Is there a will I'm not aware of? How will our children handle all this? Will they blame me for something I said, something I did or didn't do?

So many questions. It's all overwhelming. All unknown territory. Something we never planned for. How can you plan for this?

The patient says, thinks, *How can I leave her/him behind? Who will take care of her/him? How did this happen so quickly? I thought I would outlive her/him. I thought I was the healthier one. I was prepared to take care of her/him when the time came, not the other way around. She/he can't do this alone. Who will be there to help her/him? Will he/she meet someone else? Will he/she love someone else in the future? Will I eventually be forgotten by those who say they'll love me forever? Our vows were to death do us part—now I'm the one parting.*

What will happen after I'm gone? Why didn't I do this or that? Why didn't I say how much I loved her/him, how much I appreciated how much he/she had shared with me in our time together? Why did I take our time together for granted instead of seeing it as a gift? The kisses and hugs, the meals, the walks with the dogs, the trips, all the precious moments together, taken for granted.

Will I be missed? Will I still be loved? Will I be remembered? Why did I think there would always be one more tomorrow?

Fear is paralyzing, the deepest chasm of grief and one that seems insurmountable. Yet it must be traversed. The illusions must be shattered. Love doesn't live in grief and fear and guilt. It lives in hope and the memories we hold dear, the ones that make us smile, the ones that lighten our heart and tell us we still have a heart. It takes courage to let go of grief and even more to let go of the fears that seem to surround us, shouting at us every day that life is too overwhelming, too unfair, too hard. We hold on to guilt thinking it somehow justifies our suffering, but it only allows it to bury deeper into our heart.

> *At night our fear is strong. But in the morning, in the light,*
> *we find our courage again.*
> — *Ziauddin Yousafzai, father of activist*
> *Malala Yousafzai*

Grief is an unwelcome guest who settles in, trying to take up permanent residence. But we have a choice in how we let grief in and when we ask it to leave. It's a process, though not a simple one.

I once told someone who had experienced the loss of a loved one to death by suicide to let the tears of grief wash over her but don't drown in them. I told someone else to let the tears of their grief be absorbed by the beautiful memories they held in their heart of that person. I hope those words brought them a moment of comfort. As unfair and impossible as it may seem at the time, life does go on, and we have to choose how and when to re-enter a world that feels completely different to us now and forever. Life now isn't like life before, but it's to be remembered and cherished and honored, not feared.

> *Tears of grief are unique. They contain chemicals that*
> *aren't found in the more mundane droplets of moisture*
> *that bathe the eyes, as if our tears wash us free of some*
> *noxious cause of sorrow. And tonight, after crying until*
> *I am empty, I have a rare glimpse of my own interior*
> *landscape—wounds piled like tiny skeletons into the reef*
> *of conscious adult life. I am aground amid my conquered*
> *traumas, stranded as a consequence of my achievements.*
> — *Carol Cassella, best-selling novelist and*
> *anesthesiologist*

I can only imagine how difficult it must be to leave this earth knowing someone you love is still angry, still bitter, unable to forgive past grievances and wrongs of mere mortals, unable to remember all the love that was present there. Grief turned into guilt, remorse, resentment, blame, sorrow—that is its own form of cancer, untreated and left to metastasize into every part of one's life.

> *At any given moment, you have the power to say: This is not how the story is going to end.*
> *—Christine Mason Miller, author and artist*

GRIEF AND DENIAL

> *Sorrow on another's face often looks like coldness, bitterness, resentment, unfriendliness, apathy, disdain, or disinterest when it is in truth purely sadness.*
> *—Richelle E. Goodrich,*
> *American author of Smile Anyway*

I believe denial is the toughest form of grief. Denial is immune to reason. It is immune to facts. It is immune to hope. It is paralyzing. It is the deepest form of grief and the bedrock of fear for both the patient and anyone close to the patient.

> *There has to be something more we/you can do.*
> *You're not telling me/us the truth.*
> *I'll go somewhere else, see someone else, try a different treatment, try a different healer, pray more, visualize more, have more positive thoughts, try this diet, these herbs, these supplements.*

I will do anything but surrender. I will do anything except believe what you are telling me.

Who are you to tell me these things? You don't know everything. Miracles happen every day—why not me?

I did everything right.

It's not supposed to be this way. I'm not supposed to go first.

I have too much to live for.

I can fight this and I can win this battle if I don't give in.

As much as we all want to believe these things, the terrible truth is that sometimes cancer is bigger than we are. It doesn't mean we should just give up; a positive attitude, a purpose for living, incorporating things into our life that support our immune system and overall well-being are important not just for dealing with cancer but our overall quality of life. But the truth is, for many the time will come to accept the inevitable, make peace with it, and live the rest of life with purpose, love, forgiveness, and hope.

Yes, miracles do happen, but do not live there. Live in the moment that has been given to you. Be present. Be grateful you have this time to share everything you've thought, wanted to say, and wanted to do before it's taken away from you.

Oftentimes, patients have gone through their own personal grief and are now on a path toward hope. However, the family or a loved one may still be mired in grief in whatever form it's chosen to take. There is a lot of tension and sometimes anger, resentment, and bitterness all around. Grief and hope both have to be respected, unless the grief of someone else becomes detrimental to the patient's own well-being as they try to explain their own state of hope or try to support and encourage someone going through their own grief, which often results in arguments and more denial and anger.

Grief lives and thrives in the whys, the what-ifs, the if-onlys, the should-haves, the could-haves. One leads to another becoming louder and seemingly more real. There are no logical, reasonable answers to these thoughts and questions. There is only acceptance of all that is unknown and may never be known. There is only forgiveness, hope, and love in the end.

> *Before you can live a part of you has to die. You have to let go of what could have been, how you should have acted and what you wish you would have said differently. You have to accept that you can't change the past experiences, opinions of others at that moment in time, or outcomes from their choices or yours. When you finally recognize that truth then you will understand the true meaning of forgiveness of yourself and others. From this point you will finally be free.*
> *—Shannon L. Alder,*
> *inspirational author and therapist*

Grief can be a necessary and beautiful emotion if it's used to cleanse our soul and reflect on the gift we've been given instead of the loss we've suffered. No thing and no one are meant to be permanent and forever in our life. We fool ourselves into thinking we will always have what we love in our life forever. We forget that people, animals, and things are only loaned to us for a reason and for a preset time. One day we too will pass, and someone will be grieving our loss in their lives.

I don't want anyone to grieve for me. I want to be remembered joyfully for what I brought to someone's life. Grief doesn't honor me or my life. Life goes on. Capture the memories, and create new memories while you're alive. Life is meant to be lived fully, not shut down in grief that only serves a useful purpose for a brief time.

Grief held so tightly can become a terminal disease in itself. If not physically, at least emotionally. People die from the grief of a broken heart. Grief keeps them from seeing any other possibility for themselves. This is when grief becomes toxic to the body and the soul.

Grief is a very selfish emotion. Grief isn't about the one lost but the loss of our own self, how we identified and were attached to the one we lost. Grief is a self-indulgent choice. That sounds cold. We're expected to grieve in a certain way and for a certain amount of time and then get over it. I think that's cruel and unrealistic.

I choose to celebrate what I lost and be grateful I had them in my life even for a brief period of time. There is a special place in my heart where I can always revisit them and remember the joy they brought me or forgive them for the pain they caused me or forgive myself for any pain I caused them. That is how I choose to define grief: not as something debilitating but as something comforting and reassuring. Every day is a gift holding the people and things we love, and that gift is held in the heart soul.

JOURNAL

- Write what you are feeling and what you are experiencing. Be excruciatingly honest with yourself. Nothing is off-limits. Curse, scream, write all the things you are afraid to say out loud. Let your tears hit the paper. This is just for you. It doesn't have to be and shouldn't be shared with anyone.
- Sometimes grief is disguised as fear. What is your biggest fear? What would happen if it came true? How would you handle it? Shine light on your fear. Take it out of the shadows.
- How does denial show up for you and those around you?
- What guilty feelings are you holding on to but are too afraid to voice out loud? What unresolved guilts are living in you and

those around you? What would it take to let go and forgive them for yourself and others?

- What negative coping mechanisms are you using—alcohol, isolation, denial, anger, resentment, guilt? Be honest with yourself. It's OK to feel these things. Give them a voice.

- What positive coping mechanisms are you using? Is there someone you can talk to who will listen with empathy, not sympathy; compassion, not just kindness?

- What's one thing you can do today that makes you smile, gives you a moment of joy? Actively seek it out and embrace it freely and without guilt. Maybe an ice-cream cone, a ride in a convertible (with the top down, of course, if there's no lightning, stepping out into the snow and feeling the snowflakes kiss your face.

- What support do you have? Support groups, positive friends, health care professionals, grief counseling, being out in nature, meditation, mindfulness, exercise, dreaming of something you'd like to do or a new place to see, caring gently and lovingly for yourself.

- Have you talked with your health care provider about the appropriateness and potential benefit of starting antidepressive or anti-anxiety medications?

- Are you suffering in silence?

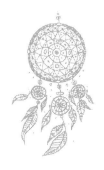

CHAPTER 3

HOPE

Birds sing after a storm; why shouldn't people feel free to delight in whatever sunlight remains to them?

—*Rose Kennedy*

At the beginning of COVID and until just recently, I experienced deep feelings of hopelessness and helplessness. There was so much confusion, misinformation, chaos, divisiveness. Where was the hope for all those who lost so much so needlessly? Where was the hope for families who were told their loved ones were dying but they couldn't be there to hold their hand or tell them they loved them one last time? Where was the hope for people who died by suicide because they couldn't stand any more pain? Where was the hope for cancer patients who were scared to death of getting COVID and dying from that before they had a chance to survive their cancer? That sense of hopeful innocence was gone.

I retired before COVID, but I can imagine how sad and frustrating it must have been for the physicians, nurses, and patients to see each other in a mask, only the eyes to convey what they were feeling, thinking—a barrier forced upon everyone for their own well-being. Lives were being lived in COVID limbo, overwhelmed by all the loss we were forced to see every day.

EMPOWERMENT OF HOPE

What is *hope*? According to the American Oxford Dictionary, as a noun hope is "a feeling of expectation and desire for a certain thing to happen." As a verb, hope is "Wanting something to happen or be the case."

For me, hope as a verb may only be wishful thinking and has no power. *I hope it rains tomorrow, I hope I get that raise, I hope I get better.* But hope as a verb can also be a prayer. It's the verbalization and manifestation of hope, the utilization of its energy.

Hope as a noun has intention, purpose, empowerment. *My hope is to experience my treatments with minimal, manageable side effects. My hope is that this clinical trial I am on not only helps me but those who follow me. My hope is my family understands, respects, and supports my decisions regarding my care.* Hope in this context is a powerful affirmation.

Hope is like a seat belt. It keeps you buckled in during the cold, scary, bumpy ride of whatever you're facing. It anchors you to the moment, keeps you steady, allows you to even close your eyes for a moment until the fear passes. It reminds you that you're still safe and being held by something stronger than yourself. You could take the ride without it, but you'd be flailing about and exhausting all your energy just trying to hold on. Hope grounds you.

Hope is a way to refocus, put things in a different perspective, and see a new or different possibility even if it's just for a moment. Sometimes just that brief moment of light is enough to pass through the darkness of fear and despair and see a glint of a different possibility. Once a seed of hope is planted, it roots itself very deeply, like a lotus flower planted in the deepest, thickest mud but able to emerge through the darkness and murkiness and bloom. From the surface, you only see the fragile bloom, but its roots go deep, anchoring it so it floats easily and steadily on the surface. This is how hope lives in me, and this is the kind of hope I try to offer others so they can plant their own lotus seed.

Hope is a gift of the heart and soul. It is available freely to anyone if they're willing to accept it. We can't fully realize the power and possibility of hope and the beauty that's waiting to be expressed until we plant that one magical seed and let it take root. We may not be able to feel or see it growing, but then suddenly, it breaks through the surface and everything is changed. Hope is my lotus flower. I have planted many, and they've changed my world and sometimes the worlds of the people around me as they plant their own seeds.

Sometimes the destructive, overwhelming power of metastatic cancer is beyond our most heart-held visualization and prayers for remission and cure. That's not a reason to forego hope. But do not cling only to hope and ignore or deny or be angry at the reality of the situation. Both possibilities must be gently held and respected.

Hope is very personal, and it should be respected, honored, and encouraged. Hopelessness is the most fatal of conditions. It kills a person's dignity and sense of purpose. Hope should never be stolen from someone no matter how impractical or impossible it may seem. Hope is as essential as breathing. It keeps the heart beating in its most natural rhythm. Hope is the vaccine against guilt and grief.

FAITH, COURAGE, AND HOPE

Hope can be a powerful force. Maybe there's no actual magic in it, but when you know what you hope for most

and hold it like a light within you, you can make things
happen, almost like magic.

—Laini Taylor, American
young-adult fantasy author

Hope is connected to faith, each dependent upon the other for nourishment, a symbiotic relationship. But what is the source of hope and faith? Is it a religious or spiritual knowing, a mindful awareness? Why is it so easily available and powerful for some people and missing for others? Can hope and faith be given by another, or is it self-generated by the heart? Is hope a source of embarrassment?

Hope lives in its own image and appears at its own calling, unannounced. Hopelessness doesn't see another day, another possibility, and this creates the opening for fear, guilt, and grief to sneak back in and sabotage everything by turning it black. Fear, guilt, and grief feed off despair, hopelessness, the unknown. Grief and fear tie the knot of hopelessness, entangled and enmeshed, unable to be freed. As they are gently untangled, each is freed of their hold, and hope is replaced.

Why does the thought of choosing hope make us feel a little more vulnerable? Are we afraid of what others will think of us, that we're being foolish, impractical, unrealistic? Or are we afraid of being disappointed and made to feel foolish if our hope isn't realized? That's not what hope is about. The fears, reluctance, and sense of vulnerability are coming from the mind, but hope comes from the heart soul.

Hope is meant to be irrational and impractical and unpredictable—all the things we're taught and told to avoid at all costs. We think our mind is the only source of our intelligence and wisdom, but our heart soul is the deeper, truer source and the one we're less tuned in to. Hope is that gentle whisper that comes from the heart soul, hoping you will pay attention and have the courage to consider what it's saying just for a moment and then to believe even when there's no proof to support what it's saying to you or trying to show you.

This is when you choose to sit with your vulnerability, let it become quiet and absorb the spirit of hope into your being. Trust yourself, suspend your doubts and fears, and allow the possibility of what hope is trying to offer you. Instead of your mind trying to dissolve hope, let hope shape your mind into acceptance. Relax and sink into your hope. It's yours alone and doesn't have to be explained or justified to anyone. It can be your own secret shared only with your heart soul who created it. Even if it doesn't actualize exactly the way your mind wanted it or thought it should be, hope always fulfills its own greater purpose in its own special way.

Faith is hope's partner, there to support you in those moments when you're feeling most afraid. It's the unseen but deeply felt presence of hope and faith that will overcome all doubt and fear and guide you through the darkest moments with their light. From my own personal and professional observations and experiences, I have noticed the power of faith when someone is facing and experiencing a possibly terminal or critical disease. Their faith may be religious or in something more powerful than themselves—a faith in the universe and the unknown, a faith in their own destiny, a faith in fate.

Faith, regardless of the source, gave these patients a sense of courage and a will to face challenges they never thought they would or could face. With faith and courage, the journey became less dark, less fearful, less treacherous, and more hopeful. They knew at some level they were not alone.

Faith, courage, and hope are powerful medicines, but they are not enough by themselves. Faith in science, in research, in health care providers, in treatment is vital. Truthfulness, trust, and openness between the provider and patient are essential. Being a cancer patient, whether on standard-of-care treatment or part of a clinical trial, is a partnership with responsibilities for all sides.

FORGIVENESS AS A STEPPING-STONE TO HOPE

Forgiveness is a powerful part of hope. Forgiveness, resentments, and bitterness cannot live together. Forgiveness is healing. Resentments and bitterness are lethal. They are each a choice.

It's easy to justify resentment and bitterness, but these negative emotions don't heal anything physically, mentally, emotionally, or personally. Forgiveness is more difficult to express, but it's actually easier and more effective for well-being than maintaining a justification for the resentments and bitterness you continue to hold on to. There is no opportunity to forgive after you're dead. Do you really want to go to your grave carrying resentment and bitterness that should have died and could have died long ago with the simple words "I forgive you" and "I forgive myself"?

I have seen families torn apart because the patient or a family member was holding on to some perceived wrong from years ago that probably could have been forgiven as a human mistake or at least forgiven as a tragic wrongdoing that bore no connection to the present. Forgiveness isn't about forgiving the perpetrator for the wrong—letting that person off the hook. Forgiveness is about freeing yourself of the resentment, bitterness, and hatred that the wrong has held over you, making you a hostage in your own life. Forgiveness is a pathway of healing, a pathway to hope, that bitterness is trying to block.

Make peace with yourself and all your shortcomings, misbehavings, wrongs committed, time lost. Forgive those who you thought wronged you. Forgive yourself for the wrongs you caused. Denial, blame, and resentment keep you stuck and unable to find the gift waiting on the other side—hope and love.

> *You only have to forgive once. To resent, you have to do it all day, everyday.*
>
> —*M.L. Sledman, author,*
> *The Light between Oceans*

ON THE BRIDGE FROM GRIEF TO HOPE

A good friend of my neighbor was diagnosed with glioblastoma multiform (GBM) on July 11, 2022. He awoke that day, according to his good friend who happens to be a retired physician, walking in circles, unable to focus, staring down to the left. He was sixty-seven years old.

Prior to this event, he had been healthy, a journalist and newspaper editor of a major newspaper in California for thirty-seven years, and a book editor. Although he was retired, this was how he identified himself—not as someone sick and out of control of his life. He had loved his job. He'd had the opportunity to interview several influential people and saw his stories headlined in the paper and read by American presidents.

Thinking his friend might be having a stroke, my neighbor drove him to a local emergency room where stroke protocols were implemented, including a CT scan. Seeing a suspicious area, the doctors ordered an MRI of his brain, which showed a walnut-sized mass in the frontal lobe. Four days later, the patient was taken to surgery for removal of the mass.

While in pre-op, scared and waiting for his surgery, wondering if he would come out of it alive or with irreparable neurologic damage, he could feel the IV fluids running down his back, soaking his gown and sheets. Obviously, something had become disconnected. He sat up and tried to stop the fluids when he was caught by a staff person and told to stop and not touch anything. She adjusted the IV and told him if he wasn't "good," he wouldn't get the surgery.

Fortunately, his physician friend was there and knew where to look for a new gown and sheets, which still had not been changed. He was caught, security was called, and he was escorted out. So now the patient was totally alone and alienated by the staff. I can't imagine anything more frightening and cruel.

Because of COVID, his partner of eighteen years, ninety years old and frail, couldn't be by his bedside. When he tried, security was again called, and he was escorted outside the hospital into sunny ninety-seven degree weather. This ninety-year-old man had to find a tree to sit under to stay cool until someone could come for him. My neighbor notified the hospital administrator of how this patient and his partner had been so mistreated. Nothing was done, not even an apology.

It took twelve days to get the pathology result—not from his neurosurgeon but as a report in his chart on his computer. Then and there he saw the diagnosis: grade 4 glioblastoma. No preparation or explanation for this devastating news. Just cold, impersonal words, a label.

For four days, he lived with the anxiety of what this diagnosis meant. He still had not spoken to his surgeon. Finally, after calling the office several times himself, he was able to get an appointment with the surgeon. His physician friend went with him and shared his outrage that his friend had been treated so inhumanely, so impersonally. The surgeon had nothing to say.

Now they had to find a radiation oncologist and medical oncologist on their own. Fortunately, they were able to get an appointment at a local, independent cancer center. From August 15 to September 20, 2022, he received fifteen minutes of daily targeted radiation to his brain with no side effects. He was started on a type of oral chemotherapy considered standard of care for GBM. He suffered terrible side effects, including nausea, sleeplessness, and fatigue.

After nine days, he decided he'd had enough, given that his prognosis with this medication was not the best. He would rather die of the cancer than suffer these debilitating side effects. The oncologist told him there was no other treatment available. He didn't mention whether a clinical trial might be available.

After doing more research, the patient scheduled an appointment with another center out-of-state considered one of the best neurological-disease treatment and research institutions in the country. They had to provide his medical records from the hospital where he had his surgery. The medical records department said that it would take ten days to get them. He strongly explained he didn't have ten days to wait; he had brain cancer and needed these records now so they could be sent to the new center. The medical records department finally relented and had them available in an hour.

He received an MRI on November 5, 2022, which indicated a recurrence of the malignancy. Not as bad as initially, a sort of pixie dust of microscopic malignant cells, but growing quickly. The patient was not surprised.

He had surgery at this center on December 15, and the cells were "scraped." He was discharged the next day with good neurologic function, no side effects, and no pain.

He is now scheduled for repeat MRIs every two months to monitor for progression or hopefully remission. Fortunately, his out-of-state center was able to refer him to a local oncologist so he wouldn't have to make those long trips. He says if he has another positive MRI, he will have no more and let life take its course. Today he feels well, his hair is growing back, he's able to perform all his activities of daily living, and he is enjoying a good quality of life. He recently went on a cruise with his physician friend, who is also his travel buddy.

He thinks he now vacillates between a little denial and peaceful acceptance. He understands the life expectancy for this cancer. He had been away from the Catholic Church since 1982 but now finds his Catholic faith to be a source of strength, comfort, and hope.

Another friend told him and his travel buddy about a retirement home for Catholic priests in Perryville, Missouri, of all places. This friend gave him a blessed medal of Our Lady of the Miraculous from this site, which he wears around his neck. He feels it's protecting him, and he can feel its positive energy. He and his travel buddy made the trip to Perryville. They described the grounds as very spiritual, healing, peaceful, beautiful, and inspiring.

He says that since he started wearing this medal and taking this trip, he feels a deeper connection to the universe, is more introspective, and is more aware of what's really important in his life—like bowling (no kidding). He has bowled independently and on leagues for the last fifty-seven years. His lifelong goal has been to bowl a perfect game. He's gotten close—299. Bowling has been how he defined himself as an athlete. It's an important part of who he is, and fortunately, he's still able to enjoy it.

Right now, he feels like he's living between a dark and cold place and one that's mysterious. Cancer has given him a gift of self-reflection and the time to just be present to his life. He has reflected upon the deepest fear he held until 1993—that he's gay. Now he sees that was a fear that didn't serve his true self, which is a beautiful, intelligent, spiritual, caring human being who is also gay. Now he also reflects on all the amazing friends he has, has always had. Some knew he was gay before he came out, and those who didn't accepted it without judgment because they love the person he is and always has been.

Because of this unforeseen and challenging experience, he thinks he may have answers to questions people haven't even asked yet. He has more insight into the world. The shades of grey he used to try to navigate have gone away. Now he has a sense of freedom he never had before.

He does not feel any less close to his partner. In fact, his partner was exceedingly distraught upon hearing of his cancer diagnosis, to the point of tears. His partner is as supportive as possible under their present circumstances, which have not been positive as of late, and will stand by him as needed as long as he is sick. They have both prepared end-of-life instructions.

He doesn't know what will happen to his partner if he dies, and he doesn't think his partner will be able to care for both of them. Still, his partner asks about his health daily. Overall, he feels his disease has separated them emotionally, but part of that is his partner's own deteriorating health since his own surgery in July, 2022.

His physician friend has pledged to stand by him. He has been totally supportive since the diagnosis without missing a single meeting or appointment, except for a few radiation treatments. He doesn't know what his life would have been like had his friend not been his voice and advocate.

The patient and the retired physician met by chance, as they were each taking a walk in the same neighborhood shortly after the patient moved there, three years before this diagnosis. Who could have known then what an important part they would play in each other's lives? The physician has been his friend, confidante, advocate, and voice in the most difficult of times. He has offered a safe space, positive support, and courageous optimism. They've not only been travel buddies on their trips, they're travel buddies on this journey. There are no accidents. We have no idea how a chance encounter may affect our life down the road, the serendipitous blessings we may be given when we least expect them but need them the most.

This patient had the worst of experiences surrounding his cancer diagnosis and initial treatment. Fortunately, this is not the norm. Hopefully, he is now on the right path, with better caregivers, and will receive the care he deserves. No one should ever have to go through what he did. No wonder patients are afraid to speak up, to ask questions, to be afraid they'll be thought of as difficult.

Every patient needs an advocate and a voice to speak up for them when they're unable to. As a patient, you deserve and have the right to be treated with respect and compassion, to have your questions answered honestly and completely, to understand your treatment plan and options. You are not there for their convenience. This is your life. You have to be fearless.

One of the biggest fears I saw in my cancer patients was not the fear of death but the fear they would lose their independence and not be able to make their own choices about what they wanted for the rest of their life, however long that might be. Hope gave them the ability and power to independently choose for themselves and be at peace with their choices.

DENYING HOPE

Light breaking through the window.
Curtains pulled to kill the hope.
Time erased, grief denied,   .
Sands of change washed away.

A friend of mine was diagnosed with the same breast cancer her mother had died of at her age (forties). She convinced herself that she was going to die the same death as her mother, even when I told her the treatments today were very different from the treatments her mother had undergone and were more successful in creating a remission. She relented and had surgery, radiation, and chemotherapy as the latest standards of care but never allowed her husband or any family member or friend to accompany her to her appointments or treatments. In her mind, she was sure nothing was going to work for her, and nothing did. Her cancer progressed.

She was very close to her only adult son and told me she wanted to take him on a trip, just the two of them, and tell him what was happening to her. She said she would do it "next year." I wanted to tell her to do it now while she was still able to travel and enjoy the experience, but I knew she wouldn't listen to me.

She died shortly after we talked, just like her mother, in her forties. We'll never know what the outcome might have been if she at least had a small glimmer of hope to hold on to and believe in, if she had gone on that trip with her son. She chose what she believed and made her thoughts and beliefs into her reality.

A seventy-year-old patient was diagnosed with stage 4 (metastatic) melanoma. She was very angry about the diagnosis, about the inconvenience treatments would cause, the commute of seventy miles each way once a week, the scheduling of the treatments. When the oncologist and I met the patient for the first time, he explained that there was currently only one standard of care treatment available, which was not very effective and had potentially terrible side effects.

A new phase 1 trial using an immunotherapy drug was offered. We outlined the trial and explained the potential side effects, risks, benefits, time commitment, and requirements for compliancy. I must admit, given her anger, resentment, and overall negative attitude, I wondered if this patient was a good candidate for this trial. After expressing her dislike of so many of the trial conditions, she signed the consent and treatment began.

From the beginning. the patient complained about her infusion time, which was scheduled in the mid-morning so there would be time for the labs, the oncologist's exam, and the infusion. The patient wanted a late afternoon appointment, which wasn't possible due to the scheduling of other patients. We explained this, but each visit resulted in the same argument.

The patient was always late for her appointments, causing other patients to be delayed. She wasn't happy if there was a wait for an infusion chair to become available, even though she was late for her scheduled appointment. Sometimes emergencies happen in the infusion suite, and there are unavoidable delays. The infusion staff patiently listened to her complaints and tried to explain all the procedures, but the anger was always there.

What could have been a tolerable and hopeful experience for the patient became one of increasing anger and negativity directed to everyone she met, including her life partner. Initially, there was a partial response, but then progression, referral to hospice, and death followed within a few months. I often wondered whether, if her attitude had been better, the outcome might have been better. At least her quality of life, and that of her partner, might have been better.

Negative emotions, stress, and anxiety can affect the immune system negatively, which could affect the response to an immunotherapy drug. Hope, positive attitude, and managing stress may enhance the effectiveness of an immunotherapy drug and just as importantly contribute to a better quality of life and overall well-being. By the way, those immunotherapy drugs are now FDA cleared for melanoma and other cancers, with very promising results and an excellent outlook for remission.

Another friend loved to make jams and jellies and always wanted to own a LeCreuset Dutch oven to cook them in. Though she could certainly afford it, she thought it was an unreasonable extravagance given her current health condition and uncertain future. She had been diagnosed with multiple myeloma, a blood cancer, a few years prior. She was handling it well—working and traveling, enjoying her granddaughter and her partner. She was still able to make those delicious jams and jellies and give them to friends, but she never bought that Dutch oven. How much better might they have tasted to us if she had? Would we have tasted more of the joy and love she had in making them in her favorite pot?

Making these condiments was part of her sense of self, something that gave her life purpose and meaning and joy. Nothing big but everything. She denied herself a pleasure that was priceless.

> *Sometimes you just need to give in to the yuckiness of the day, throw your psychic hands up in the air, and trust that tomorrow will be an improvement.*
> —Amy Shearn, author

LIVING HOPE

> *Lots of things have happened to me, and I'm glad I did what I did. You know, I was never sure how I'd be able to stand up under pressure and how I'd make decisions, and I feel good about myself for the first time in my life!*
> —Charles Schulz (Charlie Brown)

By contrast with the patient in the Denying Hope section above, an eighty-year-old patient also diagnosed with stage 4 melanoma and on the same trial had the same distance to commute but looked forward to it because he was traveling with his daughter, and the commute gave them time to talk about things even though he lived with his daughter. He always arrived on time for his appointments. He was always smiling, had a great attitude toward his treatments, and made the infusion nurses smile during his treatments.

His only request was to have a glass of wine with dinner while he was on the trial. He didn't ask for this initially, but about halfway into the trial, he asked me if it was possible. He told me his father had been a winemaker and ever since he was a boy, he'd always had a small glass of his father's wine at dinner. He asked if he could have just one small glass, because dinner didn't seem the same without it. Having a glass of wine always reminded him of his father and the great food they enjoyed together. I spoke to the oncologist, and he agreed it was a reasonable request.

One of my first patients on a clinical trial had stage 4 breast cancer. It had progressed to the point where the cancer was breaking through the skin. She still felt relatively well, but she knew her cancer could not be cured.

She had always wanted a Mercedes but didn't want a three- to six-year loan knowing she probably wouldn't live that long. Instead, she leased one on a short-term lease, so if she died before the lease ended, the car could be returned. She drove it every day even if it was for a short distance until she was no longer able to. Then her son drove her around in it with the music playing and the windows down.

One patient had been a member of the Red Hat Club for years. The members were like family to her. They were having their annual convention in New Orleans. She asked me to ask her oncologist if her trial treatment schedule could be slightly changed so she could attend. She had already bought her new red hat.

I told the doctor the clinical trial allowed for this change in schedule.

She went to the convention and returned to continue her treatments. She lived several months afterward, happy that she had fulfilled her hope and was still a participant in a life she loved. I believe she knew this would be the last convention she would attend. Knowing this, she made it the best one yet. She gave a gift to herself and to the others who attended.

Another patient loved to travel. She was seventy-four years old, with stage 4 ovarian cancer, and had beaten the odds for eight years. It wasn't easy for her, but traveling was a big part of who she was. Her former husband had been a pilot. She took advantage of every opportunity to travel while she was on the trial—either short or long trips.

She went to England with her seventy-five-year-old boyfriend, who had recently given her a beautiful aquamarine promise commitment ring. Her last trip was to Croatia, which she thoroughly enjoyed with her boyfriend. She knew the day would come when she wouldn't be able to travel, so she took advantage of every opportunity, enjoying every day she could. *She* defined her life, not cancer.

Another patient on trial knew his days were numbered. He and his family loved RVing and Labrador retrievers. Before his condition worsened and before he would eventually go to hospice, he bought a new RV and taught his daughter and wife how to drive it, back it up, and park it. He also bought a Labrador retriever puppy and taught it how to go out and fetch his morning paper. He wanted his family to continue doing all the things they had loved doing together and remember him as he lived, not as he died. That was his gift to his family.

> *A dog doesn't try to give advice, or judge you; they just love you for who you are. It's nice to have someone who will just sit and listen to you.*
>
> —*Charles Schulz (Charlie Brown)*

One of my patients bought a parrot. Even with the best of outcomes, the parrot was going to outlive her. I made a comment that parrots can live to be 100 years old. She knew that but said she had always wanted a parrot and to teach it to talk.

She made arrangements for someone to care for her parrot after her passing. The parrot gave her laughter and happiness for several months. The parrot reminded its new owner of the love her previous owner had for it every time the parrot spoke in the patient's voice.

Another patient loved golf and had played in tournaments before her cancer diagnosis. While on trial, she missed one of her treatment appointments, which was unusual for her. When we contacted her to find out why she wasn't at the center for treatment, she said she was at a golf tournament in Arizona and wasn't going to miss it since it might be her last—and it was. She did return for treatment, but she knew the truth of her ultimate outcome and chose to live the final days her way, doing what she loved as long as she could.

MISUNDERSTANDING HOPE

A different experience for a cancer patient was a young woman who had stage 3 melanoma of her arm, after having been stage 2 for six months and having a large resection of her right arm, along with lymph nodes and a full-depth skin graft. The next round of surgery left her with a very painful and minimally useful right arm. Technically she was cancer-free, but at high risk for a recurrence.

She was referred to us for evaluation of her eligibility for a new phase 1 clinical trial using an immunotherapy drug that had previously been FDA-cleared for metastatic stage 4 melanoma. The purpose of the treatment was to prevent another recurrence of the melanoma, especially a metastatic recurrence.

It was difficult for her to explain, and she was reluctant to explain to her family, friends, and coworkers, what was going on with her and why she was seeing an oncologist and receiving cancer treatment infusions and frequent CT scans when she no longer had cancer. Some people weren't aware of the seriousness of melanoma. It is a silent killer. She was well educated and having a successful professional career as an attorney.

She was extremely compliant with the demands of the trial. She experienced some side effects, which were difficult to attribute to the trial drug, as this was a first-in-human treatment for someone technically cancer-free. We monitored the side effects, which consisted of some brain fog, numbness of her right fingers, and pain in her right hip.

There is a strict process of monitoring side effects and their attribution or non-attribution to the study drug. These side effects are graded from 1 (minor) to 5 (life-threatening or death). We gave most of her side effects a grade of 1 or 2. However, these grades don't account for the emotional or professional toll on the patient.

She had been preparing to present a case to the state Supreme Court when the brain fog left her feeling less than confident to do the presentation. She delegated this once-in-a-lifetime opportunity and challenge to a coworker so the client would be represented to the best of everyone's ability—very honorable and very unselfish on her part. But this also came with another cost: she had to share with her coworkers why she wouldn't be presenting and was choosing someone else. It was embarrassing and in a sense an invasion of her privacy and a possible threat to her future career.

Because she wasn't the "typical" cancer patient people were used to seeing or thinking about, they didn't know how to respond or interact with her. Some didn't say anything, some "ghosted" her, some were condescending, some were overly optimistic in a very phony way. She looked well on the outside. How could she be sick, especially from a cancer that had been removed?

Cancer wasn't the cause of her divorce. It was a wakeup call and a mirror reflecting all that had been wrong for several years and was now irreparable. There was no connection, understanding, or support from her husband for what she was experiencing physically, mentally, and especially emotionally. Was it because he couldn't deal with it or didn't want to deal with it? Regardless, the outcome was the same—his infidelity and her further isolation and grief.

Her two daughters were young at the time, so she could only share so much with them that they would understand and not be frightened by the cancer or the pending divorce. They understood the scars on her arm and the functional limitations she was experiencing with her arm and hip. They couldn't understand her exhaustion when she had always been so active. They sensed the stress between their parents. They helped as much as they could.

The hip pain progressed, and routine scans showed rapid degeneration resulting in bone-on-bone rubbing. Her oncologist arranged for her to see a joint specialist, and once the immunotherapy treatments were done, she was able to receive cortisone shots to keep her from limping.

A couple of years after her final treatment and still having significant right hip pain, she saw an orthopedic surgeon. He recommended a total hip replacement, even though she was in her forties. Again, this was something difficult for her and the people around her to understand. Hip replacement is for old people. She had always been a runner and physically active. The surgeon strongly recommended no more running.

Now something else she loved had been taken from her. She wondered if this was some kind of divine joke. Not funny! Did the accumulating stress she was having in her personal and professional life contribute to the side effects she was experiencing? Unrelenting and unresolved stress has a very detrimental effect on the immune system.

Five years after immunotherapy treatment and numerous CTs, there is no evidence of disease (NED). She threw herself a five-year thriver party, inviting the people who had been there for her in a positive way, celebrating her divorce, her new home, and the new life she was creating for herself. Due to a prior commitment, I was not able to be there to share the joy, which I regretted.

It's still not easy for her emotionally. There is lingering grief, but now also a sense of real hope. Her daughters are doing well. Her career is going well. She has met someone who may have potential. She is learning how to be more forgiving of herself, less judgmental, more open, less controlling—not easy for any of us.

She is giving herself permission and time to enjoy life again, like planning a reunion with her friends from law school, going skiing once a week, riding her bike to the farmers market, or taking her new puppies for a walk. She is committed to creating a life she loves with people she cares about and who care for her in the most authentic, positive, supportive way.

Wanting to be part of a community and feel loved is not being needy. It is the most human of basic wants. So why are we so afraid to seek this kind of connection and feel safer being isolated, even if it makes us miserable? The most challenging love is self-love. We beat ourselves up for our perceived shortcomings and weaknesses and don't acknowledge or celebrate our strengths and achievements. We're afraid to share who we are on all levels and in all circumstances. We're negligent in taking care of ourselves and giving ourselves the things we need physically, emotionally, mentally, and spiritually, the things that make us who we are. We are afraid to embrace and nurture hope.

On December 13, 2022, Moderna announced optimism for a phase

2 clinical trial for a melanoma vaccine using an immunotherapy drug and mRNA vaccine. The patients who took the vaccine and the immunotherapy drug saw a 44 percent reduction in the risk of death or the cancer returning. A phase 3 trial is expected to begin soon.

COURAGEOUS HOPE

A dear friend of mine was diagnosed with bladder cancer in January 2018 at the age of seventy-seven. He had gone to see a urologic surgeon about a hernia repair. During surgery, the surgeon saw a suspicious area and fortunately decided to biopsy it. It came back positive for bladder cancer invading the bladder wall.

Of course, this was devastating news, and a surprise to him and his wife. They called me, and I recommended an oncologist I had worked with for several years who was actually on staff at a university cancer center where they lived. They saw him a couple of weeks later, and he laid out a treatment plan that was aggressive but probably his best chance for survival: chemotherapy plus surgery (cystectomy—removal of the bladder, which would mean he would have a cystotomy bag for urination). It was a plan they agreed with because the oncologist had explained all the risks and benefits, and they felt confident in his management of their care.

Unfortunately, my friend had a serious underlying risk factor—low platelets—which meant he was prone to easy bleeding both from the chemotherapy and the surgery. A few years earlier, a hematologist had treated him with steroids (standard of care) for this condition discovered due to a severe nosebleed. The steroid treatment was minimally successful.

Knowing this history, his oncologist recommended a new drug that he thought was promising and wanted to start him on before chemotherapy and surgery so his platelet count would improve to a safe level. However, the drug cost several hundred dollars per pill. Insurance wouldn't cover it, and the patient couldn't afford it (most people don't have those kinds of financial resources, especially someone on Social Security).

The oncologist contacted the pharmaceutical company, explaining the patient's history and his financial situation, and the pharmaceutical company provided the drug. Many pharmaceutical companies have programs to help patients in financial need. Usually the social worker at the cancer center or the oncologist can assist in this process.

In April 2018, my friend started a very aggressive regimen of chemotherapy (four months of treatment usually given over six months). Each treatment lasted four to five hours, and he spent that time talking to the other patients in the infusion suite, trying to lift their spirits. He has a great sense of humor and just makes you feel better when you're around him. After four months, he completed the regimen with virtually no side effects.

The bigger problem came in trying to find a surgeon who would do the bladder surgery, most thinking it was too risky. My friend went to three other top cancer centers in the country, and each surgeon declined to take his case, citing his age and underlying platelet complication as too risky.

He and his wife returned to their oncologist. who called a urologic surgeon he had previously worked with, explaining the situation and saying that he would manage the patient's platelets, so that shouldn't be a consideration for not doing the surgery. He added that the patient was a great candidate physically, mentally, and emotionally. The only hitch was that the surgery had to be done within thirty days of completion of the chemotherapy for best results, and time was ticking.

The surgeon agreed to take the case and rearranged his surgical schedule to meet the time requirement. My friend came through the surgery with no side effects, accepted the ostomy bag, and he and his wife learned how to care for it.

This case strikes me for several reasons. There was honest communication among everyone involved. The patient was an advocate for his own care, and there was teamwork among everyone involved—the oncologist, the surgeon, the ostomy nurse, and the patient. No one fell through the cracks.

The story continues. In September 2020, during COVID, while taking a walk in his neighborhood, my friend started feeling a burning in his throat and thought it was from the smoke from the neighboring wildfires. He walked home and told his wife, who immediately drove him to the ER. They were there within minutes, and they were told he was experiencing a massive heart attack and needed to go to surgery immediately.

He informed them of his platelet situation. They did the appropriate bloodwork, which confirmed a very low platelet count. They suggested steroids (the usual treatment), and he told them it wouldn't work, but he had his platelet meds at home and they should call his oncologist to verify. His wife went home to get the drugs.

The ER called his oncologist to verify and started him on the medication. He was admitted for observation, and about three days later, his platelets were above normal and he went to surgery for a quadruple bypass. Again, a knowledgeable, involved patient and teamwork led to successful treatment.

As soon as he was able, he got out of bed and started walking the halls of the hospital several times a day, knowing that the more he could be up and moving, the sooner he could go home. Since this was during COVID, his wife couldn't be with him in his hospital room. She would stand outside his window so they could see each other. What he didn't know was that when she left the hospital, she allowed herself to cry and feel scared and helpless but not hopeless. He left four days after the surgery with no side effects.

Today, four years after his cancer diagnosis with no evidence of disease, two years after open heart surgery (no complications), and at eighty-one years of age, soon to be eighty-two, he is playing eighteen holes of golf every week with his friend. His goal is to have his golf score match his age, and he's almost there.

He gets up every morning, takes care of their two cats, takes a walk around the neighborhood, goes out to lunch with his wife, and has an occasional glass or two of wine, or champagne, at home. One of his mantras during all these challenges was "this too shall pass." He has told himself this during every difficult time of his life. His other philosophy is "Life is life. If you think you won't, you won't. If you think you will, you will. It's all in the cards." He wants to be there for his wife who has been by his side through all of their challenges. And he says his cats need him. He thinks he'll live to be 100. I think so too.

This patient is a great example of the powerful combination of education, hope, faith, attitude, positive support, open and honest communication, and proactive medicine. This isn't always the case, but it can and should be.

Also, these patients didn't let cancer define them. They continued to be who they had always been and live their lives as best they could for as long as they could, or they would create a new life, one they loved. That was their hope as a noun. That hope became their reality. When some did pass, it was with grace, dignity, and a knowing they had lived their life as fully and authentically as they could, with nothing left undone or unsaid.

Life is not a dress rehearsal. There are no retakes. Life doesn't wait for you to find the perfect script, memorize your lines, find your inner essence, and have a killer audition. Life says, *You're up, let's see what you got.*

> *The secret of a full life is to live and relate to others as if they might not be there tomorrow, as if you might not be there tomorrow.*
>
> —*Anaïs Nin, diarist, essayist, and novelist who kept a diary from age eleven until her death in 1977 at the age of seventy-three, providing profoundly explorative insight into her personal life and relationships.*

CANCER IS A TEAM DISEASE

Being a team player in your case means speaking your concerns, asking questions, being educated, and being an active participant in your care. It also requires showing respect and gratitude for all those who are trying to save your life, ease your suffering, and maintain as good a quality of life as possible. Remember, all the health care providers you come into contact with are there by choice, are on your side, and want the best possible outcome for you. When they go home, they are still thinking of you and if there's more they can possibly do.

HAPPINESS AND HOPE AND CANCER

> *What makes night within us may leave stars.*
>
> —*Victor Hugo, French Romantic writer and politician*

Halloween was a big, happy event at our cancer center. All the clinics, departments, and infusion suites had different themes, and all the staff dressed in fun costumes. The patients loved it.

One of my patients who had recently gone on trial but who had experienced previous Halloweens at the center dressed up in a big guinea pig costume and visited the other patients, telling them she was the guinea pig on a phase 1 clinical trial. Everyone loved it, and it brought her such happiness knowing she had made other patients laugh and for a moment forget, including her. I have a picture of her in her costume with me. I love it.

Happiness doesn't seem to go with cancer. How can you be happy with cancer? Yet I've seen many people with cancer who are happier at this point in their lives than they were before their diagnosis. They don't take anything for granted anymore. They make the most of every moment. They are totally present to their life, the people around them, their surroundings. They feel a deeper kind of love and connection to themselves and others than they've ever felt before.

They seek out relationships that are supportive, nurturing, and hopeful, and disregard those who want to bring them down by telling them how awful it is that they have cancer or who don't want to be around them at all—shunning them and trying to make them feel fearful, guilty, or powerless over their disease. People with cancer can find the space that brings them happiness and live in that space without explanation or excuses. Yes, happiness is possible in these moments. Happiness brings hope, and hope brings happiness. Happiness is no longer about accumulating things, making good impressions, or comparisons to others. Happiness now is about acceptance, gratitude, awareness, and love. It's about celebrating life every day. This is the gift cancer gives, wrapped in the ugliest paper.

Buy yourself flowers or whatever else you like and surround yourself with things of beauty, things that make you smile, things that bring you a moment of joy, things that bring you hope no matter how unreasonable it seems. We should all do this for ourselves every day regardless of the current state of our health.

Don't wait for your funeral to buy flowers. Don't wait until you can no longer enjoy the things you love, the things that make you you. Continue to discover new things about yourself and your life. Savor every moment. Remain a participant in your life. Hope isn't about practicality. You can't control life, and you can't let life control you. You can only be in life.

> *There are things that our souls metabolize to be healthy. We need beauty, we need truth, and we need goodness.*
> —*John Mackey, cofounder of Whole Foods*

CANCER AND HOPE TODAY

Today's cancer is different from the cancer of years ago. Treatments are available today that weren't available even a few years ago. They are more effective, saving more lives, prolonging lives with a better quality of life for the patients. Resources are available today that weren't available before. New research is ongoing every day for better treatments and better drugs to alleviate negative side effects.

NEW HOPE IN TREATMENTS
AND PREVENTION

> *And life is eternal and love is immortal, and death is only a horizon, and a horizon is nothing, save the limit of our sight.*
> —*Bede Jerrett, English Dominican friar and Catholic priest, noted historian and author*

There are many hopeful things happening for cancer patients right now. According to the American Association for Cancer Research, eight new anticancer medications were approved by the US Food and Drug Administration between August 2021 and July 2022, as well as ten previously approved medications that have been expanded to treat other types of cancer. These new drugs, like immunotherapy drugs that use the body's own immune system to kill the cancer cells and targeted therapies that attack specific cancer cell mutations to kill them, are less toxic and more effective than previous treatments. Some are used in combination with chemotherapy drugs. Side effects are recognized earlier and managed more effectively.

Immunotherapy drugs are successfully treating metastatic melanoma and certain lung cancers. Targeted therapies are zoning in on specific cancer cells, disabling them without harming the body's own good cells. Genetically engineered creation of CAR-T cells (chimeric antigen receptor T cells taken from the patient's own blood) are designed to kill specific cancer cells. In recent studies, nine out of ten people with acute lymphoblastic leukemia (ALL) whose cancer didn't respond to other treatments or whose cancer came back had full remission with CAR T-cell therapy.

Various vaccines are currently in clinical trials to treat early- and advanced-stage cancers or prevent cancer in certain high-risk patients. In the future, there may be a blood test to diagnose cancer in its earliest stage. This could make screening more accessible and more affordable, and detect cancers earlier when they're more successfully treatable.

In 2022, there were more than 18 million cancer survivors living in the US, equivalent to 5.4 percent of the population, the AACR report found. Fifty years earlier, there were just 3 million cancer survivors.

There are now very successful preventive measures available. Quitting smoking, of course, is one of the most successful in the prevention of lung cancer and certain oral cancers. Although this has been known for decades, smoking is unfortunately increasing in certain populations.

Yearly gynecologist exams, monthly breast self-exams, mammograms, colonoscopies, testicular and prostate exams are very effective in finding early stage, treatable cancers. HPV vaccines are available for boys and girls, men and women, ages eleven to forty-six to prevent cervical cancer and some oral and anal cancers caused by the human papilloma virus (HPV). Genetic testing, such as BRCA screening for the early detection of genetic mutations that could determine a woman's risk for breast and/or ovarian cancer, is readily available through a geneticist. Men should also have a BRCA test if they have a female relative positive for the BRCA gene mutation, as this puts them at higher risk for breast cancer as well.

Semi-annual dental exams can detect early oral cancers. Yearly skin cancer checks with a dermatologist, especially in high-risk areas of the country, can detect early skin cancers, including melanoma. Something as simple as wearing sunglasses and using sunscreen can help prevent skin cancer. Prevention is an important weapon against cancer. Prevention is always a preferable option over treatment.

Early cancer screenings must become more accessible for underserved populations, especially people of color who are at higher risk for certain cancers. Insurance companies must become more flexible about approving screening tests for younger populations who are becoming a higher risk for certain cancers. Screenings cost a lot less than treatments.

SUPPORT AND CANCER

There are things you can do to help your overall well-being while living with cancer:

- Exercise. Get out of bed even if you don't feel like it.
- Go for a walk, be outside, and enjoy nature.
- Put on some upbeat music and dance like nobody's watching.
- Sing like nobody's listening.
- Visit and explore a new place.
- Get a mani-pedi.
- Maintain positive social connections.
- Keep a gratitude journal and enter at least one thing every day.
- Meditate even if it's just for a few minutes at a time. There are several meditation sites online. I personally like guided meditations, as they offer a subconscious sense of well-being and mindfulness in addition to the actual meditation.
- Go to a museum or art gallery, or a zoo, especially a petting zoo or an aquarium—someplace where there's life and no thoughts of death, a place where people are happy, smiling, and creating. It's OK, and necessary, to let yourself feel happy and smile for a moment.
- Be aware of your diet and include more beneficial changes, like a Mediterranean diet, small frequent meals, eating when you feel hungry, eating what tastes good to you, sucking on lemon drops and ice chips, and taking anti-nausea prescription meds if needed. Speak to your cancer center's dietician or nutritionist for recommendations and support.
- Seek out a legitimate local or online support group for your particular cancer type. Educate yourself about your cancer, appropriate treatments, and how other people have dealt with their cancer in the most positive way.
- Communicate with your health care professionals—we are not mind readers. Ask for what you need.

We need people in our lives with whom we can be as open
as possible. To have real conversations with people may
seem like such a simple, obvious suggestion, but it involves
courage and risk.

—*Thomas Moore, Irish author,*
poet and composer

CLINICAL TRIALS

Lastly, learn about clinical trials. They are the future for successful cancer treatment. They are very regulated and monitored. Patient safety is always of the utmost concern, not only for the pharmaceutical company conducting the trial but the institution and health care providers implementing it.

Eligibility requirements to enter a trial are very strict. Not everyone is eligible to go on a trial. A person on a trial is not a guinea pig. No modern drug today would be available without the people who bravely chose to participate in a clinical trial. New treatments are being discovered. Cancer-fighting drugs like immunotherapies and targeted therapies were not available even a few years ago. For more information, visit www.clinicaltrials.gov.

According to the *Journal of the American Medical Association*, the University of Washington has recently completed a ten-year phase 1 clinical trial of a DNA vaccine for HER2 positive breast cancer. Patients for a phase 2 clinical trial are currently being recruited.

A phase 3 clinical trial for metastatic melanoma conducted in the Netherlands shows promising results, as reported in the December 7, 2022 issue of the *New England Journal of Medicine*. It uses immune cells harvested from the tumor itself. These cells are called tumor-infiltrating lymphocytes (TIL). Those who got TIL therapy had a 50 percent reduction in disease progression and death compared to those who were treated with standard-of-care immunotherapy treatment, and 20 percent of TIL patients had a complete remission. Future clinical trials are being considered using TIL therapy for other solid tumors. Hopefully, this trial will become available in the US.

Trials are being conducted at cancer centers around the world to learn more about cancer cell biology and genetics and more effective treatments.

> *There is no medicine like hope, no incentive so great and no tonic so powerful as expectation of something tomorrow.*
> *—O. S. Marden, American inspirational author who wrote about achieving success in life and founded SUCCESS magazine in 1897. He was a New York City lawyer, a leader of the Legal Aid Society, and a president of the American Bar*

A clinical trial is a combination of things patients don't understand—why vital signs have to be taken before an EKG and an EKG before the blood draw and they all have to be taken in a certain way at a certain time; why all side effects, even those that seem minor or not related to the treatment, have to be taken seriously and reported immediately; why they have to meet strict eligibility requirements to go on a trial when they're thinking they just want to live regardless of the cost, the side effects, the potential ineffectiveness of the trial, anything for one more chance. *Just give me the damn drug* they said when I had to tell them they weren't eligible for the trial because of a negative lab test or their physical inability to do everything the trial required or some other criteria that couldn't be met.

They thought all they had to do was sign the consent, not even wanting to read it. *Just give me the pen.* I was the one who told them, *No, you have to read it, read it with your family, write down your questions and concerns so we can discuss them before you sign.* Going on a clinical trial may be voluntary, but you must sign an informed consent, and I as the cosigner of the consent have to know you understand in a way that you know what you're signing up for.

Some patients who were willing to sign the twenty-, thirty-, forty-page consent form without looking at a single word would later, after reading it, have questions and fears that could be honestly addressed and answered to their comfort level. Many didn't understand all the scientific nuances, and some were fearful of all the potential side effects they might experience. Some after reading would reconsider and choose to not go on the trial and let the disease take its course. I honored both decisions and was their advocate when others may be urging them to do anything possible to "cure" the disease inside them.

Some patients were at peace with where they were on their journey, and others wanted to climb another mountain if it was there. Agreeing or not agreeing to go on a clinical trial is educational, emotional, and the most personal decision a person will ever make, especially for a phase 1 trial where the outcome is hopeful but unknown. But there would be no phase 2 trial if there weren't people courageous enough to be part of a phase 1 trial, and no phase 3 trial without a phase 2 trial, and no drugs for any condition without a clinical trial.

People who choose to be part of a clinical trial are heroes, and they should be respected and treated as such. That was how I tried to meet each patient. I was humbled that they trusted me as well as the rest of the clinical trial team. I always wanted them to know that what they were doing was brave, honorable, and overseen scrupulously, and their well-being, dignity, and voice were always honored.

Human clinical trials are not guinea pig lab experiments. They are taken very seriously because scientists, researchers, oncologists, nurses, and pharmacists know what's at stake for the individual patient and for humankind by their choosing to be part of a clinical trial. For me, the biggest challenge of a phase 1 clinical trial in particular was how to impart hope while also being honest about the possible results or lack of results. The patients trusted their oncologist who was leading the trial, and they trusted all the staff that were administering the trial. It was a partnership: patient, oncologist, research nurse, trial staff.

These were the most challenging years and the most rewarding years of my professional career. I truly admired these patients and learned as much from them as hopefully they learned from me.

JOURNAL

- What is your one hope just for today?
- What is one thing you are grateful for today?
- What is one positive thing you can do for yourself today?
- What is one thing you've always wanted to do? What's keeping you from doing it?

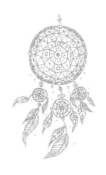

CHAPTER 4

LOVE

Only people who are capable of loving strongly can also suffer great sorrow; but this same necessity of loving serves to counteract their grief and heals them.

—Leo Tolstoy, author

Some families are torn apart by a cancer diagnosis. Others find a deeper love, a new kind of love, not the heated physical love that may have initially brought them together but the deeper emotional and spiritual love, a gentler love, a more understanding love. A love of empathy, not sympathy. A love of compassion, not just kindness. A love of forgiveness and authenticity.

EXPRESSIONS OF LOVE

Love makes your soul crawl out from its hiding place.
—Zora Neale Hurston, novelist

My twenty-eight-year-old patient arrived at the cancer center with her three boys, ages eight, six, and five. She had no one to take care of them. Her husband, the children's father, had recently been deported to Mexico because of a minor traffic violation. She was here to start day one of the clinical trial, which involved drinking three small bottles of a powdered drug mixed with water.

I saw the anxiety on her face and the fear on the faces of the boys. Children weren't allowed in the clinic rooms or the treatment suites. I told them to wait for me while I went to the pharmacy to get the bottles of study drug. I found a quiet conference room and brought them in, boys huddled around Mom.

This was the time of Harry Potter. I told the boys these bottles had a magic potion and they could help me mix it and give it to their mom so she would feel better. I gave each boy a bottle, took off the cap, handed them the water, and told them how to mix it.

Soon they started smiling and everyone was laughing. I told them they were magic wizards. Each boy handed his mom the bottle he had so carefully prepared. She drank trying to hide her tears and telling her boys how proud she was of them and how much she loved them. I'm sure the medicine tasted better to her.

She took home the bottles for the next several days' doses and told her boys they could prepare it for her at home. Now they were active participants in their mom's care, and it didn't seem so scary.

> *Magic exists. Who can doubt it, when there are rainbows and wildflowers, the music of the wind and the silence of the stars? Anyone who has loved has been touched by magic. It is such a simple and such an extraordinary part of the lives we live.*
>
> —*Nora Roberts, author*

Glioblastoma multiform (GBM) is a cancer of the brain or spinal cord. As it progresses, it affects speech, movement, mood, and memory. Unfortunately, there currently isn't a cure for GBM. Treatments focus on removing or shrinking the tumor to reduce symptoms.

The first step is surgery to remove the tumor (craniotomy), followed by radiation and chemotherapy. If surgery isn't an option due to the patient's poor health or the tumor's location, radiation and chemotherapy or targeted therapy may control the tumor. A new treatment involves a wearable device that sends low-intensity electric fields (TTFs) to the tumor through electrodes on the scalp. TTFs disrupt cancer cells, preventing them from multiplying and growing. This treatment may be provided after chemo–radiation is complete.

One GBM patient had been through surgery and chemo–radiation, but the GBM progressed. He was in a wheelchair and unable to speak, but there was still a twinkle in his eyes, especially when he looked at his wife, and he could still smile at her. She was a retired nurse, and he had been a professional photographer and musician.

He and his wife chose to go on a phase 1 clinical trial, as this was the last option available to him. Because there was a long infusion time and multiple blood draws and EKGs to be performed, the patient was given a private room with a bed in the infusion suite so he would be able to rest and be comfortable during the long day.

As soon as I got him in the bed, his wife crawled in too. She curled up next to him as she had every night of their fifty-year marriage. They lay together during the long day and brought each other peace and comfort.

Every time they came for his treatment, they lay together, she talking softly and gently to him, music playing in the background. Better than any drug. The love between them was evident, and it had grown in spite of his terrible disease and all they had endured.

So close that your hand on my chest is my hand, so close
that your eyes close as I fall asleep.
                    —*Pablo Neruda, poet and winner of 1971*
                                     Nobel Prize in Literature

Another GBM patient on this same trial and being cared for by another research nurse told her how much he loved McDonald's pancakes. Knowing he was going to be at the cancer center most of the day like the patient above, on her way into work she stopped at McDonald's and got him two orders of pancakes so they would be there when he arrived. He was so happy when he saw them and enjoyed every bite. Something seemingly so small but so thoughtful made his day. Pancakes gave him a sense of normalcy.

JOURNEY OF LOVE

A brief history of a young, vibrant, beautiful woman who would become my future patient.

She was born in 1960, the youngest of four children. This was a time when smoking was accepted and cool. Ads were everywhere. Actors were smoking in movies and on TV, even *The Dick Van Dyke Show*. Most of her family members, including her parents, smoked.

She started smoking at sixteen and smoked about three-quarters of a pack per day. She started cutting back on her cigarette usage in September 2009, several years after her mother had passed away from small-cell lung cancer. She got down to six cigarettes a day.

In February 2010, she wasn't feeling well and was able to quit entirely after an urgent care visit. She told her family smoking could destroy their lives and to think about all the people that were important to them and how those people would feel if they didn't exist anymore. They didn't listen.

In 1973, this patient's mom had been experiencing a persistent cough. When her husband came home from work and saw her slumped in a chair, he took her to the ER, where she was diagnosed with a collapsed lung. She was diagnosed with breast cancer in 1974 or 1975 and had "chopped up" surgery and radiation treatments for two to three weeks. The mom was a very private person and didn't share much with her family, especially her youngest daughter, who was only fourteen at the time.

In early 1989, still smoking, my patient's mom started experiencing shortness of breath and was feeling bad. She had a chest X-ray, which showed scarring from the collapsed lung, but no diagnosis of cancer was made until 1992. She was told there was nothing they could do except buy some time.

She initially didn't want chemotherapy but relented and received treatment from April to July. She eventually went into the hospital, where hospice care was offered. The family chose to bring her home with outpatient hospice and an overnight nurse so her husband could get some sleep. My patient started working part-time instead of full-time so she could be with her mother and help with her care. She and her mom had been very close, going shopping and out to lunch, mother-daughter dates.

Although the hospice nurse had given her instructions and phone numbers to call, she wondered what she would do if her mom died while she was there alone. It was a very frightening thought. Her mom died in September 1993 at age fifty-nine, just nine and a half days after coming home from the hospital. All the family was there.

During all those years, my patient's father had been very supportive, but his wife told him to go to work and not worry about her, she was OK. She was a very independent person.

In January 2010, my future patient was out shopping for Super Bowl Sunday. She started feeling "crappy" but thought it was due to the exertion of shopping. In February, her fatigue worsened. She called her primary doctor but couldn't get an appointment for three weeks.

Several days later, but before her primary doctor appointment, she went to urgent care. They listened to her lungs, said they sounded OK, and prescribed a seven-day course of antibiotics. She continued to feel worse and saw her primary doctor, who told her the antibiotics she had been given weren't strong enough. The doctor prescribed something stronger that she should take for ten days.

She continued to feel a heaviness in her left chest. Her primary told her it could be fluid or chronic obstructive pulmonary disease (COPD). She returned to her primary a third time in April, who wanted to refer her to the pulmonary clinic. The patient demanded another chest X-ray before seeing the pulmonologist. Her primary reluctantly relented and gave in to her so she would have some "peace of mind, dear."

After the X-ray was completed, the technician asked her why she had come in for the X-ray, and she explained how she had been feeling. He told her it was good she came in. Her primary called her that evening and said there appeared to be a mass in the upper left lung. A CT was ordered.

She saw a pulmonologist, who explained everything to her in a way she could understand without being condescending. He told her he was 99 percent sure it was lung cancer. She didn't feel any shock hearing this news. She had suspected it for some time.

He wanted to show her the scan and the mass, but she was hesitant. Her husband looked at it and then she did. It was a five-by-seven-centimeter mass below her collarbone. Now it was real.

She asked what her options were. He told her surgery was a possibility, and she asked if it could be done the next day. Unfortunately, that wasn't possible due to the pre-op things that needed to be done before surgery. She had a PET scan and brain MRI, pulmonary function test, and biopsy right away. The biopsy was positive for non-small cell lung cancer (NSCLC).

She met with the cardiothoracic surgeon May 24, who confidently and patiently explained the surgery, which was scheduled for that next week, June 2, 2010. He made her feel secure. She felt a sense of relief from being proactive and knowing a plan was in place.

When she tried to talk with her sister about her diagnosis, the sister had some "choice" words for her, saying *I'm not going to screw up my life taking care of you*. No one except her husband wanted to talk to her about her diagnosis, as if talking about it would make it too real. They would quickly ask her how she was doing, and she would say fine—the dutiful question to ask and the expected answer to give to make everybody feel better.

The day after surgery, she was out of bed and walking. She wanted to walk more but had to wait for an available walker. She was discharged four days later.

At home, she started walking on an old treadmill she had bought in 1994. She did laps around the house, walking up and down her stairs three times a day, gradually increasing to five times a day and then ten. She had two separate post-op chest X-rays, which looked good.

She was referred to a medical oncologist July 15, 2010, for prophylactic chemotherapy to kill any free-roaming cells. He sat down and explained everything to her in a very compassionate, patient, humane way. He told her not to surf the Internet about her disease, because there was too much information that was wrong and possibly dangerous. She immediately felt a sense of trust and connection with him.

He told her she would be "put on the clock," and if there was no recurrence in two years, her treatment could be considered a success. She received three cycles of chemotherapy, the last on September 20. She had some slight nausea and fatigue but overall tolerated it well.

In December, she went back for a three-month checkup. A CT was done that showed the left lung looked good, but there were two small spots on the right lung, one in the upper lobe and one in the middle lobe, possibly an artifact.

In March, she had another CT, the last day her favorite oncologist would be on staff at the cancer center. This CT was positive for cancer. She was shocked at this unexpected news. She'd had no indication of anything being wrong with her right lung.

She was referred to a radiation oncologist for a consult. He explained to her that radiation could possibly be performed on the one spot high up in her upper lobe, but he wouldn't be comfortable delivering radiation to the other, as it was too close to her heart vessels. She asked what her options were. He recommended chemotherapy.

She was referred back to a new medical oncologist at this center who was not "warm and fuzzy" like her previous one. This oncologist coldly told her she couldn't be cured, would die from this, and treatment would only "buy her time," echoes of her mother. The patient felt shock and irritation at the doctor's callous, dismissive demeanor.

She was scheduled to begin a combination of three chemotherapy drugs ten days later based on the pathology of the cancer cells. She had another CT and brain MRI. She was told she would have treatment every three weeks for four to six cycles and would definitely lose her hair within two weeks of the first cycle. In preparation, she went shopping for scarves. Her husband and sister went with her to buy a wig.

When her hair started to fall out, she measured out three inches from her scalp and cut her beautiful brown hair. She at last felt in control of her body and the decision she was making. Her sister had wanted her to have a hair-shaving event, but she said no. This was too intimate, too personal to be shared with others.

When she lost more of her hair, she asked her husband to shave her head, but not too close. She lost her eyebrows. She developed a rash that was irritated by the wig and cotton scarves. She bought silk scarves and baseball hats, which reflected her own personal style, wearing them even at home. She would shape and define her new identity.

The first chemo treatment lasted six and a half hours. They sped up the second treatment slightly to shorten the infusion time. She experienced an infusion reaction, with pain in her chest and back, and the skin on her chest turned a bright red. Another IV was started, vital signs were taken, and she was given an antihistamine. It was a scary moment for her and her husband, who always accompanied her.

They lengthened the rest of the cycles, which went without incident. She found it less stressful to walk around the infusion suite instead of sitting in a chair for several hours.

Her weight dropped to ninety-eight pounds. She experienced nausea and got antinausea meds. The meds improved her appetite. She craved Panda Express beef and BBQ ribs even though the nutritionist had told her she shouldn't eat spicy foods. These were the foods that tasted good to her and she could tolerate and enjoy.

There were nights during this time she would wake up and think *you have cancer*. She found it difficult to sleep the week before a scheduled scan from anticipating it and a week after the scan waiting for the results. She asked for an anti-anxiety medication.

She and her husband started reading various publications and stories from cancer survivors about the positive things they had done during the course of their disease. A common thread was movement and exercise. They bought a new treadmill. She was so excited about getting it that this was the first thing she shared with her oncologist when she saw her for follow-up.

After a few treatments, her oncologist called her and asked if she was having tingling or numbness in her fingers or toes, which she was to a small degree. The doctor changed her regimen to one of the drugs instead of three. Her last treatment was in November.

She had a CT scan, which showed no improvement. Again, the patient asked what her options were. The oncologist had been investigating a phase 1 clinical trial and thought it would be of benefit to her.

This is when we met. I explained the trial consent to her, which she signed. I explained she had to be off her previous treatment for one month so the drug was out of her system and began scheduling the required studies needed prior to treatment to confirm eligibility. She was scheduled to begin in January of 2012. The study consisted of two targeted oral therapy drugs taken every day for twenty-eight days. After two cycles, there would be another CT scan. She and her husband began planning a trip to Maui.

On March 10, 2012, she had the CT that showed a 25 percent increase in the size of the tumors. Since the treatment wasn't effective for her, she was taken off the trial as mandated by the study. No one stays on a trial that isn't benefiting them.

Again she was referred back to the radiation oncologist. Again she asked what her options were and if another surgery could be an option. At this point, she felt she had nothing to lose. The radiation oncologist told her he thought that could be a reasonable option, and she was referred to a different cardiothoracic surgeon at the cancer center for evaluation.

That surgeon told her the original surgeon should have never done her first surgery—that this surgeon was an "idiot." He said he would have to be convinced by a lot of other people that surgery was a good option for her. He wasn't saying no, but he wasn't saying yes.

He showed no compassion toward her. She felt scolded and dismissed. She was confident he wasn't the right choice for her. How could she trust someone with that kind of attitude with so much at stake? Literally her life.

She retrieved her medical records and contacted her original surgeon. He asked why she hadn't returned for her follow-up visits with him after the original surgery. She explained no one had told her she had any appointments. Unfortunately, she had fallen through the cracks. She told him about her visit with the other surgeon. He reassured her he was confident this was a reasonable surgery for him to perform. She was immediately scheduled for surgery that week, March 30.

This surgery was tougher for her. There was more pain. Staples were used to lift the right middle lobe to the chest wall. A wedge resection was done, with clean margins obtained. She was in the hospital eight days with a chest tube. The fluid didn't seem to be draining adequately, so she was hooked up to wall suction, which meant she couldn't leave her room for her walks until two days before her discharge.

A bronchoscopy was done three days after the surgery. During the procedure, her surgeon came by to see the images on the camera for himself. He saw she was in pain and hyperventilating and told her her lungs were inflamed. Two days before her discharge, she began feeling better and was able to get out of the room and walk the halls. By the eighth day, she was ready to go home.

She saw her surgeon in his office on Monday and Wednesday of the next week for chest X-rays. He told her the chest X-rays showed fluid, and the middle lobe was not lifting. It was determined that the fluid needed to be removed, which was done by a guided CT. The most painful part for her was the actual pulling out of the fluid.

She thought she would stay in the hospital one night, but she spiked a fever, so she had to stay three. She finally went home on oxygen.

In June, she was exercising and started coughing. She coughed up a little blood containing a staple. She contacted her surgeon, who immediately saw her. While at the office, she coughed up another staple. He told her these were stabilizing staples and though it was rare to have them be coughed up, it wasn't anything to worry about. At home, she coughed up one more. She now has three staples in a plastic cup.

On July 3, she and her husband left for Maui.

In the fifth year of her cancer diagnosis, she was referred to another oncologist, as the previous one had left the practice. Before she saw him, she pulled up her records on the computer in the patient portal and saw an addendum to her November CT scan. It indicated calcifications in the lymph node, concerning for a recurrence, and she should be re-evaluated.

She asked the oncologist about this. He stated he had read the addendum before she came into the clinic. He told her they would start her on a new FDA-cleared immunotherapy drug for lung cancer and then do another CT and, if necessary, a biopsy.

She told him she wanted the biopsy first and was told this wasn't the standard protocol. She said she didn't care about protocol. She wanted the biopsy. Fortunately, her insurance agreed to it. She was referred to another pulmonologist who biopsied six samples. She received the results seven days later—active cancer of the aorta-pulmonary (AP) window.

Again, she asked what her options were. She was told surgery would be extensive and was referred back to yet another new oncologist and the original radiation oncologist. The oncologist started her on the immunotherapy treatment in April 2017, delivered twice a month. Radiation was started in combination with the immunotherapy—ten treatments Monday through Friday for two weeks. She finished October 30.

In November, she had a PET scan that showed no evidence of disease. She was on the immunotherapy until January 10, 2018 (sixteen treatments in total). She has been in remission ever since.

In June 2021, she saw another new oncologist after her usual follow-up scan. He explained that there was a big shadow on her right kidney, which was not a stone. She was surprised. She'd had problems with her left kidney but never her right. He was concerned it could be renal cell carcinoma and scheduled an MRI. Fortunately it was a cyst, not cancer.

During this MRI, a lump was seen on her right breast. An ultrasound was done and then a biopsy, which showed papilloma cells (noncancerous). She was referred to a breast surgeon in November 2021 for consideration of a lumpectomy. The surgeon didn't think this was necessary, since a microchip had been implanted and she would be followed every six months on future scans. In April 2022, the ultrasound showed no evidence of disease.

This was a tortuous journey and one that is not yet over. She experienced the best and the worst from health care providers but was never intimidated or coerced into something that didn't seem right to her. She made her own informed decisions.

Overall, she is doing remarkably well. Her beautiful hair has grown out and is now curly. She still has some tingling in her fingers and toes and some knee pain. Her energy level isn't quite what it used to be. Her brother and sister-in-law have become more supportive since her second diagnosis of lung cancer.

It has been a very long journey, and the thought of another cancer occasionally crosses her mind. She has rarely complained or said *why me*. Her husband has been by her side every step of the way, there for every appointment, every hospitalization, every treatment. Her husband has recently been diagnosed with a slowly rising PSA (possible prostate cancer indicator), so now he's being monitored by a urologist, and she's there with him for his appointments.

I am certain her positive attitude, tenacity, strong will, and proactive decisions, along with her husband's support and love, have made a positive difference for her. She will continue to be monitored every six months and then hopefully every year and lead a long, productive, purposeful life.

Everything has its wonders, even darkness and silence, and
I learn, whatever state I may be in, therein to be content.
—Helen Keller

LIFE AND LOVE INTERRUPTED

A friend of mine, a mathematician, recently shared with me his experience of having testicular cancer when he was a younger man. In the summer of 1980, he went through a month of extreme tiredness and loss of appetite. A gastroenterologist ran a series of tests but found nothing. The conclusion was that it must be a spastic colon. Months later, on December 3, 1980, at age 36 and never married, during a visit to his urologist, a lump (or pathology as the urologist called it then) was discovered. He was scheduled to have surgery to remove the testicle on January 7, 1981, a lifetime of waiting for him and a date he'll never forget. The urologist told him not to worry about it. He'd be fine. Easy for him to say. Scheduling was backed up because of the approaching holidays.

He was living on his own at the time, in a rather new city in a home up against the mountains with amazing views of the mountains and the city lights below, running marathons, having a successful career that he loved with an innovative technology company. A perfect life.

He had just met a woman who would later become his wife although at the time the relationship was rather on again, off again. He was uncertain how to tell her what was happening with him. When he did share the diagnosis with her she was stunned and not quite sure how to respond, like most people when they hear the word "cancer". She was supportive but did not fully understand the complexity of the disease. She would visit when she could to help him with routine household things.

Some people, especially at that time, looked at someone who said the "C" word with the unspoken but obvious thought on their face "are you dying, are you going to die?" He could see it on their faces. They didn't know what to say and stumbled to try to say something positive.

He had a previously scheduled business trip, a briefing at the Pentagon with a Navy Admiral, to discuss the future of hypersonic missiles over cruise missiles. He said the Admiral tried to intimidate him by his questioning of the proposal, but he thought, *"I'm dealing with cancer, this is nothing. You can't intimidate me"*.

After the trip he went to visit his oldest sister in New York State who happened to be an Operating Room nurse. She arranged for a second opinion which confirmed the diagnosis. He asked her not to tell their other three sisters or his father. His mother had died a terrible death due to lung cancer at age 56. He had two uncles who had died of throat cancer at age 50. He knew if his other family members knew of his diagnosis, they would think he would be dying soon too and he did not want to put them through that anxiety.

When he returned home, he had a chest X-ray which revealed spots in both lungs, most likely positive for metastatic disease although a biopsy wasn't done. His urologist referred him to an oncologist. His sister wanted him to return to New York to see an oncologist she knew and be treated there. He chose to stay in his home. His oncologist told him if he didn't have cancer he'd be in perfect health. Ironic but not especially comforting.

In February 1981 he started chemotherapy. Treatment for metastatic testicular cancer was in its infancy at this time. The oncologist explained all the possible side effects. He thought since he was otherwise so healthy, he wouldn't have any of the side effects. He was terribly wrong. He was started on a combination of a platinum drug and cytotoxic chemotherapy drugs. The platinum drug was administered in the hospital overnight and then the other two drugs were administered, and he was sent home. This was to be repeated every three weeks. Simple. Not.

He experienced what seemed like all the side effects the oncologist told him were possible. He was living alone and barely able to walk from his bedroom, down the hall to the couch, and then collapse, staring up at the ceiling thinking it needed to be painted. He had severe and frequent vomiting, all his teeth hurt, he lost his hair, had numbness in his feet and fingers. He called his oncologist who told him to come to his office. A friend drove him. He was barely able to get out of the car but refused a wheelchair. He walked to the office building, rode the elevator up to the third floor and walked into the doctor's office where he saw other bald-headed patients. Until recently he could still recall the smell of that elevator which immediately caused a wave of nausea.

When the doctor saw him, he immediately got a wheelchair and had him admitted to the hospital across the street. He was in the hospital for three months receiving treatment. He was able to leave one day every three weeks to go home. His side effects worsened with uncontrollable physical shaking of his body. His weight dropped from 150 pounds to 100. The oncologist told him they weren't sure if three, four or five treatments would be the most successful as they were still trying to determine the appropriate dosage. Balancing the benefit of the drug versus the risks of the side effects. Sometimes more isn't better; it's just more toxic. He received four courses of treatment. His oncologist decided to skip the last treatment and told him "We'll watch you". The good news was that the metastases to his lungs had disappeared. Looking back, he thinks he was on the front line of cancer treatment for testicular cancer.

The hospital had a cancer board which included his urologist and oncologist. The Board's suggestion was to remove all the lymph nodes along his spine and neck. His urologist, oncologist and he rejected that idea as being too extreme given the real possibility of impotence. He received a CT scan every month, then every three months, then six months and then yearly. He was told if he was disease free for three years, they would consider him okay.

He called a friend who worked in the oncology division of the NIH (National Institute of Health). Not telling him he had cancer; he asked his friend what the life expectancy was for someone with testicular cancer. He didn't tell him it had metastasized to his lungs. His friend said about 40%, with metastases about 25-30%.

Today testicular cancer is curable and treated successfully in 95% of cases. If treated early, the cure rate rises to 98% without a loss of sexual function. The standard of care now for testicular cancer is surgery, radiation therapy, chemotherapy and possibly high dose chemotherapy and stem cell transplant all depending upon the extent and stage of the cancer.

One and a half weeks after his discharge from the hospital and his return home, a longtime friend flew into town to visit. At that time, you could meet passengers at the gate. His friend walked right past him, not recognizing this thin, bald-headed man. He had to call out his friend's name. Being a polite host, he wanted to show him around town. They went hiking in the mountains. Bad idea. His friend helped him back down the trail.

He was back to work within five to six months even though he could have stayed away longer. He missed what he had done for so long and wanted to get back to a "normal" life.

Since he had no appetite and was having difficulty eating, his friends brought him marijuana to smoke, the first the size of a cigar. He had never been a smoker so had never inhaled. After a quick course in how to inhale he learned how to smoke the marijuana. It did allow him to eat a ham sandwich for the first time although he still couldn't taste it.

Six to eight months after his treatment he had an ultrasound of his abdomen area which showed a shadow. He was in the middle of a multi city business trip when his doctor tracked him down. He wanted to complete the rest of the trip, but the doctor strongly recommended that he come home. *"You won't enjoy the rest of the trip anyway."* Both the urologist and oncologist wanted to see the repeat ultrasound for themselves which was scheduled a few days later and they agreed it was nothing.

He decided to go back to New York to see his family. In retrospect it was too early. They noticed his hair loss and the bruises on his arm from the IVs. He made excuses to keep from telling them the truth. One of his sisters told him if he had some terminal disease that he wasn't telling them about she would piss on his grave.

Years later, after his father had passed away, at a gathering of family and friends in his small hometown, a friend came up to him and commented on his cancer. The room became silent. His family looked at him waiting for an explanation. Now, the secret was out. He had no idea how his friend had known. A cancer diagnosis seems to have its own underground communication system.

In November 1985 he married his fiancé, the love of his life. He had hesitated to marry after his diagnosis not knowing what the outcome would be and not wanting to leave her a widow. But she persisted. She has been by his side all along. He decided to cut back on his business travel and travel only three days a week instead of weeks at a time. He wanted to spend more time with her and enjoy their home and life together. He retired in 2001, having made a significant contribution to the company before and after his cancer.

He says his philosophy became "save for retirement but live now". In October 1998 he bought a red Corvette convertible which he still has. He is living a very good and very satisfying life, enjoying his retirement in the most personally fulfilling way, maintaining contact with some of his former co-workers. Although several years have passed, he still has residual side effects from the treatment such as numbness in his feet, manageable reminders of his journey.

He says he has become a bit of a hypochondriac. He worries if something feels "off", if he feels a lump, if something doesn't seem right. He wonders what if it comes back or a different cancer occurs. How long had he been unaware of his testicular cancer, how he got it, why he got it"? It could happen again. Cancer is always at the back of his mind as it is for most cancer survivors. He's learned that if something feels really wrong it is the patient's responsibility to be persistent in tracking down the cause.

Starting as teenagers, men should do a monthly self-testicular exam like women do a monthly self-breast exam. This should be done after a hot shower or bath, so the skin is relaxed.

GUIDED JOURNEY OF LOVE

Rhabdomyosarcoma (RMS) is a rare childhood cancer. The orbit of the eye is the most common primary orbital malignancy in children. It is often seen initially by an ophthalmologist after a patient has developed symptoms such as pain, eye drooping, eyelid swelling, a palpable mass, and later blurred vision. Today, prompt diagnosis can save the life of the affected individual.

Unfortunately, my patient developed this cancer, at the age of five, long before successful screenings and treatments were available. Both eyes were removed, which was the standard of care up until the 1960s. He functioned very well for years, beating the odds, as the mortality rate at the time was approximately 70 percent.

The patient had had eight service dogs since his blindness. He told me he used to have German shepherds, but as he got older, they became too strong for him, and they walked too fast, so he was given Labradors.

He was married. His wife was legally blind but was able to see shadows and ambulate with a white cane. She said she didn't want a service dog because she "didn't get along well with dogs."

He developed a soft tissue sarcoma in his fifties which metastasized to his lungs. He received chemotherapy, but the tumor progressed. A phase 1 clinical trial was available involving an oral drug taken for four days every two weeks. Starting on day five, he would receive an injection of a drug that would increase the white blood cells, as the study drug reduced the white blood cell count, making the patient susceptible to infection, which could be life-threatening.

These injections had to be drawn up into the syringe from the medication vial and given at home by the patient in alternating sites once a day for eight days after taking the oral drug. We wondered how this could be done, since neither he nor his wife was capable of doing it. We needn't have worried. We were able to prescribe home health care, and a nurse came each of the eight days and administered the injection. He never missed one. He never missed a clinic appointment either.

Before going on the trial, he had come to the cancer center for his chemotherapy treatments with his latest service dog, a beautiful male black Lab. I met the dog for the first time when the patient came to be evaluated for the clinical trial. The dog knew his way around the cancer center better than some humans. He knew when he came in the front door to go to the check-in desk, then to the lab, then up to the third floor to see the oncologist, and then to the fourth floor for treatment. I thought this was amazing.

I asked my patient how the dog knew to do this—if the patient counted steps for each place. He said no, the dog just knew.

We looked forward to every visit of our patient and his dog. They both gave us a sense of hope and relief from the stress and anxiety we often felt. The dog seemed to know we were there to help his partner, lying quietly next to him.

When I retired, the patient was still on the trial and doing remarkably well. His dog was still by his side, guiding him every step of the way. The drug has not yet been cleared by the FDA for standard treatment.

> *The opposite of loneliness is not togetherness, it's intimacy.*
> —*Richard Bach, author*

KINDNESS

A recent study of four hundred cancer patients, family members, oncology clinicians, and staff conducted by Leonard L. Berry, University Distinguished Professor of Marketing, Mays Business School and Senior Fellow, Institute for Healthcare Improvement, Texas A&M University, showed how six types of kindness can improve cancer care:

- deep listening
- empathy
- generous acts
- timely care
- gentle honesty
- support for family caregivers

These acts seem so obvious yet so difficult to implement into a daily practice. We can all be practitioners of kindness and share these qualities with each other as part of our everyday lives.

Cancer centers are busy places—from the lab, to radiology, to the clinic and the infusion suite. Patients must navigate each of these without a lot of guidance from the staff, who too are overwhelmed by the number of patients they must see in a very limited time. Trying to get from one place to another and waiting at each place to be seen creates patient anxiety before the patient is even seen. Staff anxiety grows as they get further behind in their own schedules because the schedule doesn't allow for unforeseen events or the need to spend extra time with a patient to explain something life-changing. Each delay leads to another delay. So these six areas of kindness fall by the wayside—not intentionally, but by the rigid structure of the system.

Many cancer centers are now trying to restructure themselves to provide services that incorporate the whole patient and the family and caregivers. They are beginning to understand that all parts of the patient are interconnected, and when one area is affected, all are affected.

> *To be fully seen by somebody, then, and be loved anyhow—*
> *this is a human offering that can border on miraculous.*
> *—Elizabeth Gilbert, author*

TIME

None of us knows when we're going to die or exactly how we're going to die. It may be cancer, it may be a car accident, it may be trauma, it may be a heart attack or heatstroke or COVID, or tragically, even suicide. I've known people who have lived with cancer for several years and then died of something totally unrelated. I've known seemingly perfectly healthy people who died in their sleep with no indication anything was seriously wrong when they went to bed.

No one wakes up in the morning or goes to bed at night thinking they're going to die that day or that night. If they did, they would have said all the things they wished they had said, done all the things they thought they would always have time to do. They would have been more fearless in their life. They would have been more generous with themselves and others. They would have lived life with grace and forgiveness. And yet we all will die someday, and much of it is out of our control and often unexpected.

Life is precious. We've heard that thousands of times, but rarely do we live our life with that thought in the forefront. We always think we'll have one more day, just one more. We tell ourselves *I'll do that tomorrow.* We tell ourselves *they know how much I love them, I don't need to say it again.* Or *I forgot to kiss my wife, my husband, my children goodbye this morning; I'll do it when I get home.* And then that time, that precious gift, never comes.

> *What greater thing is there for two human souls, than to feel that they are joined for life—to strength each other in all labor, to rest on each other in all sorrow.*
> —*George Eliot (Mary Ann Evans), English novelist, poet, journalist, translator, and one of the leading writers of the Victorian era*

We get caught up in the minutiae of everyday life, trying to do more, get more, be right, prove a point, win an argument, play mind games with each other, one-up each other with a better car, better job, bigger house, better school, more money. We're afraid to be authentic, vulnerable, and honest with ourselves and others. We hold forgiveness for ourselves or others as a sign of weakness and bury it inside. We don't take a moment to receive the gratitude waiting to be shared with us or to give away the gratitude we're feeling, because it may come to be expected and, after all, there's only so much that can or should be given away. *If I give away too much, I'll have less for myself, which I may need later, so I'll hold on to it until I'm sure I don't need it.*

Don't be defined by your disease. Be defined by your life, every moment of it, and share it without regret or explanation. Share it with joy and love. You are still you, and you may be surprised by how much more of you there is. Express your love, your uniqueness, your innate purpose for the life you were blessed to live. Don't live for your eulogy. Live for this very moment and the next and the next until there are no more, and then hopefully your last breath will be one of gratitude and love.

> *The most authentic thing about us is our capacity to create, to overcome, to endure, to transform, to love, and to be greater than our suffering.*
> —Ben Okri, Nigerian-British poet and novelist.

I enjoy wine, and I receive daily emails about new wines from different wineries around the world. I received one today from Tattoo Girl in Washington State, a wine I had never heard of before. The label pictured a beautiful tattooed woman. According to the description, "the winemakers are celebrating the wine drinker—those who are bold and authentic in their actions, free in their conversations, and excited to celebrate life's beautiful moments." I think that's a great way to live life, with or without wine, with or without cancer.

Life messages often come to us in unexpected ways and from unexpected sources. I bought Tattoo Girl wine and enjoyed its essence. By the way, I have two small tattoos that I got before they became pop fashion.

One small one at the nape of my neck is an ancient Rune symbol for the infinity and eternity of spirit and soul. My life partner has the same one on the nape of his neck. We got them together.

Don't go to your grave, or the crematorium or mausoleum, with things unsaid, things undone, forgiveness not bestowed, love not expressed, joy not felt. Don't leave the people in your life wondering *what if, how*, and *why*. There are no easy answers. It may be difficult to say and do the things you know in your heart are the right things to say and do, but that's what courage is about. How better to live the final days of your life while not knowing when that may be? Today is the day to make things right, not just for you but for them—a beautiful gift given and received.

The giving of love is an education in itself.
—*Eleanor Roosevelt*

As a research nurse, I intentionally made the time to be with my patients, especially during their most stressful times—signing a consent, starting a new treatment, performing the numerous blood draws and EKGs, being told their cancer had progressed and they would have to come off the trial. Or being there when they were told the cancer had not progressed or, even better, there was no evidence of disease. Tears shed.

Cancer isn't only a physical disease; it's an emotional, mental, and spiritual disease as well. The total patient and the family must be cared for. A gentle touch, a moment to hug, an encouraging word, a look into the eyes lets the patient know they are still human, they are still alive, they are still seen and heard, and that's what everybody needs and wants in life.

ONE LAST WORD

This book is also about listening—particularly about listening to someone who is dying. I mean really listening. Listening to what's said and what's left unsaid but understood. Listening to the silent spaces between the spoken words. For both, this may be very uncomfortable.

You may think it's easier to not have this conversation, but trust me, it's not. This conversation is absolutely essential for you both. The person dying knows they're dying, and as much as you may wish this wasn't true, you both know it. So embrace it.

I know that sounds strange, but if you can embrace the truth of this reality, you have an opportunity to learn things you would not have learned any other way, and the person dying has the opportunity to share those things with you that they feel are the most important and honest. This is a time for honesty. It's not a time for guilt or finger-pointing.

Being honest doesn't mean being cruel. It means accepting the fact that you were both human beings who had shortcomings, work undone, and words unsaid. And now is the time to cut through all the crap and be real with each other in the most compassionate, empathetic way you can.

When you are really listening, you're not doing anything else, and you're not thinking about anything else. You're present to the other person. You're quiet inside. You're looking into their eyes and really seeing the human being there, not just the role they played in your life. You're not looking at your mother, your father, your spouse, or your child. You're seeing, maybe for the first time, the pure spirit of the person in front of you. And that's a gift you should cherish for the rest of your life.

We're all dying. Some of us are just more aware of it. Every morning when we awaken, there is no certainty that we will return to go to sleep that night. But every day we miss the opportunity to tell someone we love them; to tell them who they are for us in our lives. We think they know. We think we'll always have tomorrow to tell them. But we may not.

I've worked with patients who were in the process of dying my whole nursing career. The hardest thing to see is someone who knows they're dying but is trying not to know so their family or loved ones won't have to think about it or deal with it. So much goes unsaid between them. Some are unwilling to speak these last words, but you can see in their eyes what they would like to have said. And the most unfortunate part of this is that the family and loved ones will never hear those words, never have those memories to recall and give them comfort.

As painful as it may be at the time, when it's over, it's those words and memories of that final time spent together that offer the most comfort to everyone. There were dreams and secrets that died with my mother that I'll never know and may have made a difference in my own life.

The daughter of one of my patients arranged to video her mom as her mom shared her life story—where she was born, why she loved the Smoky Mountains, how much she enjoyed being a teacher, where she wanted her ashes spread. Those images and words would now live after her departure.

Learn to listen with an open heart. Most of us listen with our egos. We're defending ourselves in our minds while the other person is speaking. We're judging the other person. Quiet your ego and listen to what's really being said, not what you think is being said. As you listen, don't think about being right. Don't think about what you're going to say, or not say, next. This conversation is not about you but it is *for* you, no matter how difficult that may be for you to understand in this moment.

When you're talking to someone who's dying, look past their illness, their injury, their pain. See their spirit in its purest form. Their spirit is not the illness or the injury or the pain. Their spirit is not dying—it's transforming. And if you look closely, and if you're truly present, you can witness the transformation, which is beautiful and peaceful. Honor this gift that has been given to you. Some of the most meaningful life lessons I've ever learned have come from being with someone who is dying. The dying can teach you how to live.

PASSING

I remember patients who died, and I miss them and mourn for their families. I also remember patients who lived a good quality of life for a long time after receiving a new kind of treatment or procedure because they were brave enough and altruistic enough to go on a clinical trial for their disease. I remember being in the operating room when a transplant patient received the donor kidney they had been waiting months or years for, and how the donated kidney pinked up and began to produce urine when the last clamp was removed. But I also remember the deceased donor who so generously donated their organs when they passed so others could live; or the unselfishness of the living donor to give a gift of life.

Life is full of sadness, loss, love, and miracles. Life doesn't come with a money-back guarantee or exchange for a better-fitting one. We're each on our own path, our own journey, no matter how short or long it may be. But we have the power to choose how we will live while we're on this path, and no one can ask for more than that. Choice is the gift we're given in this life.

> *There isn't time, so brief is life, for bickerings, apologies, heartburnings, callings to account. There is only time for loving, and but an instant, so to speak, for that.*
> *—Mark Twain*

The heart, the beginning, the first heartbeat, the last heartbeat. What happens in between? The heart is always there—joy, loss, love, isolation, betrayal, forgiveness, lightness, heaviness. Heart is the harbinger of our past, present, and future, yet so ignored, until it is finally silenced with so much unsaid, not done.

But does the spiritual heart live on in a new creation of energy, and where does it go? What is the real energy of the heart? It's not just electrical, a bunch of atoms and molecules bumping into each other. What is the essence of the heart, and how do we let it emerge into its fullness? How do we love and embrace our own heart and all its passion and possibility and beauty? As our bodies are made of breath, flesh, bone, and blood, our souls are made of courage, faith, truth, and love, which are eternal.

The good heart, the full heart, my heart. Embraced, loved, shared. This is what I want. This is what was created in me at that first heartbeat and will live on after the last. My hope.

You can only lose something you love. If you haven't lost something in your life, you haven't loved something in your life.

> *New beginnings are often disguised as painful endings.*
> *—Lao Tzu, Laozi, ancient Chinese*
> *philosopher and writer, reputed author of*
> *the Tao Te Ching, founder of philosophical*
> *Taoism, and a deity in religious Taoism and*
> *traditional Chinese religions*

Intimacy and real love aren't only about the physical. Intimacy is an authentic embrace, a knowing smile, an encouraging word, time shared, being totally present to one another without compromise, judgment, fear or restraint.

*If ever there is tomorrow when we're not together, there is
something you must always remember. You are braver than
you believe, stronger than you seem, and smarter than you
think. But the most important thing is, even if we're apart,
I'll always be with you.*

—*Christopher Robin, Pooh's Grand Adventure:*
The Search for Christopher Robin, A.A. Milne

Love is meant to heal.

Help me to heal and release the hurts others have caused me and hurts I may have caused others.

Love is meant to renew.

Help me to renew my enthusiasm for life.

Help me to see opportunities and possibilities instead of problems and disappointments.

Love is meant to create a sense of safety and security in each area of life.

Help me to find completion in each aspect of my life.

Love is meant to inspire with its power.

Help me to do that of which I am most afraid.

Help me to do that which I think I cannot do.

Help me to do that which I am called to do.

Help me to create hope where there is doubt.

Love is meant to be fearless in the face of fear.

Help me to discover the courage lying within me.

Love is meant to unveil immortality.

Help me to feel the energy of the soul that never dies.

Help me to leave a footprint in the universe, one of love that others will want to step into and follow.

Love is meant to bring inner peace and joy and hope.

Help me to open my heart so it may be shared.

Love is meant to harmonize differences and celebrate uniqueness.

Help me to open my mind and heart to acceptance.

Love is meant to bring me closer to God and my own True Self, the Heart Soul.

Help me discover and live this higher, truer plan for my soul so I may serve.

JOURNAL

- How do you define love in your life?
- What have you discovered about love since your diagnosis?
- How do you express love to and for yourself?
- How do you express your love toward others?
- How do others express their love toward you?
- Do you feel heard?
- How do you listen to others?
- How do you listen to your own inner voice?

AFTERWORD

There is no such thing as a "good" cancer, a "small" cancer, a "harmless" cancer, a cancer that will go away by itself. Screenings are vital for everyone. Know the possible warning signs of cancer; know what's normal and what's not normal for your body.

Speak up for yourself. Make lifestyle changes. If you smoke or vape, quit. Wear sunscreen and sunglasses when you're outside. Incorporate more fiber, fruits, and vegetables in your diet and less sugar and saturated fats.

Do monthly breast self-exams. Engage in physical activities you enjoy, especially outside. Even a few minutes helps. Get a pet and let it get up on the couch and sleep in bed with you.

Obviously, everyone is different, as is each disease. You may experience all of the symptoms below for a particular cancer, a few, different ones, or none at all. You know your body. If something feels new or different, can't be explained, or you just have that feeling that something isn't right, contact your health care provider immediately.

Early diagnosis is crucial. Don't live in denial, saying it's nothing, that it'll go away, that you'll wait and see if it gets worse. No news is not good news. If you feel your health care provider isn't listening to you and is dismissing you because "what do you know," find another provider.

I had a pearly pink, scaly area on my calf. I thought it was nothing because it didn't look like any of the signs of skin cancer I was familiar with. I kept watching it and noticed it was growing very slowly. I went to my dermatologist who said she didn't think it was a cancer because it didn't look like it. But she fortunately decided to take a biopsy just to be sure.

It was a basal cell skin cancer. She removed it, obtained clean margins, and it hasn't returned. Although basal cell skin cancers are rarely metastatic, it could have grown into something much more serious if left unattended. Now I have a skin check by my dermatologist yearly or sooner if there is something suspicious.

POSSIBLE EARLY CANCER SIGNS AND SYMPTOMS

Melanoma (ABCDE):
- asymmetry
- borders (uneven)
- color other than brown or black for a mole
- diameter greater than 1/4 inch
- evolution (change in color, size, shape, or other)

Colon
- change in bowel movements
- abnormal stool quality such as thinner stool, change in color, evidence of blood
- rectal bleeding (bright red or black tar-like stool)
- abdominal discomfort or pain, bloating, cramps

- nausea and vomiting
- loss of appetite
- weight loss
- unexplained fatigue
- anemia
- shortness of breath

GI (gastrointestinal)
- abdominal pain or discomfort
- nausea and vomiting
- loss of appetite
- fatigue or weakness
- bleeding (vomiting blood or blood in stool)
- unexplained weight loss
- early satiety (unable to eat a full meal)

Breast (women and men)
- new lump in the breast or armpit
- thickening or swelling of part of the breast
- irritation or dimpling of breast skin
- redness or flaky skin in the nipple area or breast
- nipple discharge other than breast milk, including blood
- pulling in of the nipple or pain in the nipple area
- any change in the size or shape of the breast
- pain in any area of the breast

Cervical
- vaginal bleeding either after intercourse, between periods, or post-menopause
- abnormal vaginal discharge (heavy or with foul odor)
- pain during intercourse

- vaginal itching or burning
- pelvic pain
- lower back pain or abdominal pain
- abdominal bloating
- frequent urination
- pain and swelling in leg
- unexplained weight loss
- decreased appetite

Ovarian

- abdominal bloating or swelling
- early sense of fullness when eating
- unexplained weight loss
- fatigue
- pelvic or back discomfort or pain
- change in bowel habits, such as constipation
- frequent urination

Lung

- worsening or lingering cough
- coughing up blood
- chest pain
- shortness of breath
- constant fatigue
- unexplained weight loss

Oral

- persistent mouth sores that don't heal
- persistent mouth pain
- lump or thickening in the cheek

- white or red patch on the gums, tongue, tonsil, or lining of the mouth
- sore throat or persistent feeling that something is caught in the throat

Prostate
- interrupted urination
- urge to urinate frequently
- frequent nighttime urination and bowel movements
- painful urination
- blood in urine
- urinary incontinence
- lower back or groin pain
- deep, aching hip pain

Testicular
- A lump or swelling in either testicle.
- A feeling of heaviness in the scrotum.
- A dull ache in the lower belly or groin.
- Sudden swelling in the scrotum.
- Pain or discomfort in a testicle or the scrotum.
- Enlargement or tenderness of the breast tissue.

Although you may feel embarrassed by finding one of these symptoms of testicular or prostate cancer do not hesitate to see your primary physician or urologist. Don't let fear stop you from being diagnosed at the earliest possible, treatable, stage. Do not think it's nothing or that you'll wait to see if it goes away.

Pancreas

- jaundice (yellowing of the skin and whites of the eyes)
- light color stools
- dark urine
- pain in upper or middle abdomen or back
- unexplained weight loss
- fatigue
- poor appetite

Lymphoma

- lymph node swelling in neck, armpits or groin
- unexplained fever
- weight loss
- excessive sweating
- shortness of breath
- itching
- rash
- fatigue

Leukemia

- Fever or chills
- Persistent fatigue, weakness
- Frequent or severe infections
- Unexplained weight loss
- Swollen lymph nodes, enlarged liver or spleen
- Easy bleeding or bruising
- Recurrent nosebleeds
- Tiny red spots on skin (petechiae)

Don't be terrified of cancer. Don't become paralyzed by it. Be a proactive partner in the management of your cancer. Become educated through reputable sources; education is power. Seek out positive and appropriate support. Find a provider with whom you can establish a partnership for your care, a provider who sees you as a human being, not just your disease.

The human body and the human spirit are miraculous gifts that we'll never fully understand, nor should we. They are given to us to accept, honor, love, and embrace in whatever form they've chosen for us. Be grateful for all that you are, all that you've been given, all that you've endured, and all that you've sacrificed to live this life with purpose and grace.

Life is a mystery. Life is a miracle. Life is a gift in whatever form it takes, whatever journey it travels. There are no guarantees. We can only see where we think we are and maybe the next step to take, not knowing where that one step may take us, what door may open for us.

At the end of my life, my hope is that I am remembered as someone who loved and was loved; who was kind, empathetic, and compassionate; who forgave; who shared wisdom and a life full of unforgettable experiences. My hope is my life is celebrated in joy and laughter and not mourned in grief and heaviness and regret.

> *All of the rocky and metallic material we stand on, the iron in our blood, the calcium in our teeth, the carbon in our genes were produced billions of years ago in the interior of a red giant star. We are made of star-stuff.*
>
> *—Carl Sagan, American astronomer, planetary scientist, cosmologist, astrophysicist, astrobiologist, author, and science communicator.*

RESOURCES AND RECOMMENDATIONS

WEBSITES

Clinical Trials: clinicaltrials.gov

American Cancer Society: www.cancer.org

St. Jude Research Hospital: www.stjude.org

Breast Cancer Research Foundation: www.nbcf.org

Be the Match (bone marrow and blood stem cells donation site): www. bethematch.org

Lymphoma and Leukemia Society: www.lls.org

American Lung Association: lung.org

The Breast Cancer Site (for free, click to fund mammograms for under-served women): thebreastcancersite.greatergood.com

Ivy Brain Tumor Center at the Barrow Neurological Institute: ivybrain-tumorcenter.org

BOOKS

*I think books are like people, in the sense that they'll turn
up in your life when you most need them.*

—Emma Thompson, actress

Emperor of All Maladies: A Biography of Cancer by Siddhartha
Mukherjee, MD
Between Two Kingdoms by Suleika Jaouad
Becoming Earth by Eva Saulitis
The Artist's Way by Julia Cameron
Let the Whole Thundering World Come Home by Natalie Goldberg
On Death and Dying by Elisabeth Kübler Ross, MD
Tuesdays With Morrie by Mitch Albom
On Living, Kerry Egan, hospice chaplain
Brighter by the Day: Waking Up to New Hopes and Dreams by Robin
Roberts
The Book of Awesome by Neil Pasricha
*Mindful Medicine, 40 Simple Practices to Help Healthcare Professionals
Heal Burnout and Reconnect to Purpose* by Jan Chozen Bays, MD,
pediatrician and ordained Zen teacher

MUSIC

*For me, singing sad songs often has a way of healing a sit-
uation. It gets the hurt out in the open into the light, out
of the darkness.*

—Reba McEntire, singer-songwriter

"I Hope You Dance," Lee Ann Womack

"Because You Loved Me," Celine Dion

"Blackbird," The Beatles

"Easy Like Sunday Morning," Lionel Richie

"Desperado," The Eagles

"Just the Way You Are," Bruno Mars

"This Is It," Kenny Loggins

"Iris," Goo Goo Dolls

"The Living Years," Mike and the Mechanics

"Some of Us Are Brave," Danielle Ponder

"Best Day of My Life," American Authors

"Forever Young," Rod Stewart

"Rainbow," Kasey Musgraves

"Hero," Mariah Carey

"Born to Be Wild," Steppenwolf

"Kiss the Rain," Billie Myers

"You're Beautiful," James Blunt

"I Just Want You To Know Who I Am," Goo Goo Dolls

"I Will Always Love You," Whitney Houston

"Broken and Beautiful," Kelly Clarkson

"Memories," Maroon 5

"I Just Called to Say I Love You," Stevie Wonder

"Try," Colbie Caillat

"See You Again," Carrie Underwood

"True Colors," Cyndi Lauper

"Chasing Cars," Snow Patrol

"Say You, Say Me," Lionel Richie

"The Climb," Miley Cyrus

"If I Could Turn Back Time," Cher

"Live Like You Were Dying," Tim McGraw

"Lift Me Up," Rihanna

"Peace Train," Cat Stevens

"Shower the People," James Taylor

"Stairway to Heaven," Led Zeppelin

> *Look up at the stars and not down at your feet. make sense of what you see, and wonder about what makes the universe exist. Be curious.*
>
> —Stephen Hawking